Social Dance

about the author

Myrna Martin Schild is Assistant Professor of Health, Physical Education, Recreation and Dance at Southern Illinois University at Edwardsville. She has taught Social Dance for more than two decades at the university, junior college, high school and junior high school levels. She and her husband were both trained as ballroom dance instructors by Arthur Murray Dance Studios and regularly partake in ballroom dance for recreation and exercise. They have entered swing dance contests on the local, regional and national levels.

Professor Schild has engaged in a variety of professional activities of the state, national and international levels of Health, Physical Education, Recreation and Dance with the American Alliance (AAHPERD) and the International Council (ICHPER). She has taken trips around the world to research physical education and dance and has found the presence of social dance in most of the countries visited.

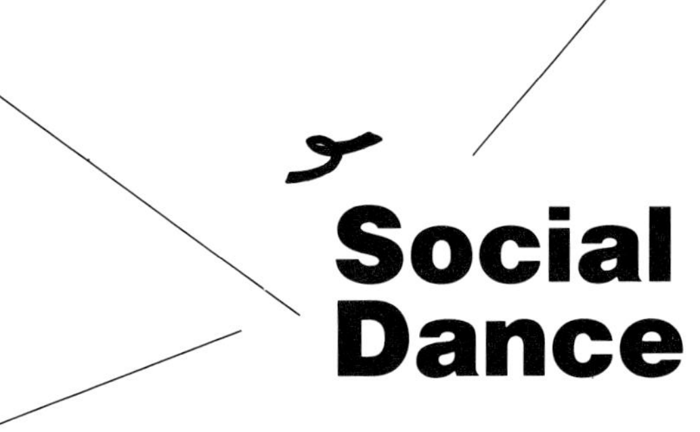

Social Dance

Myrna Martin Schild
Southern Illinois University
at Edwardsville

wcb
Wm. C. Brown Publishers
Dubuque, Iowa

Consulting Editor

Aileene Lockhart

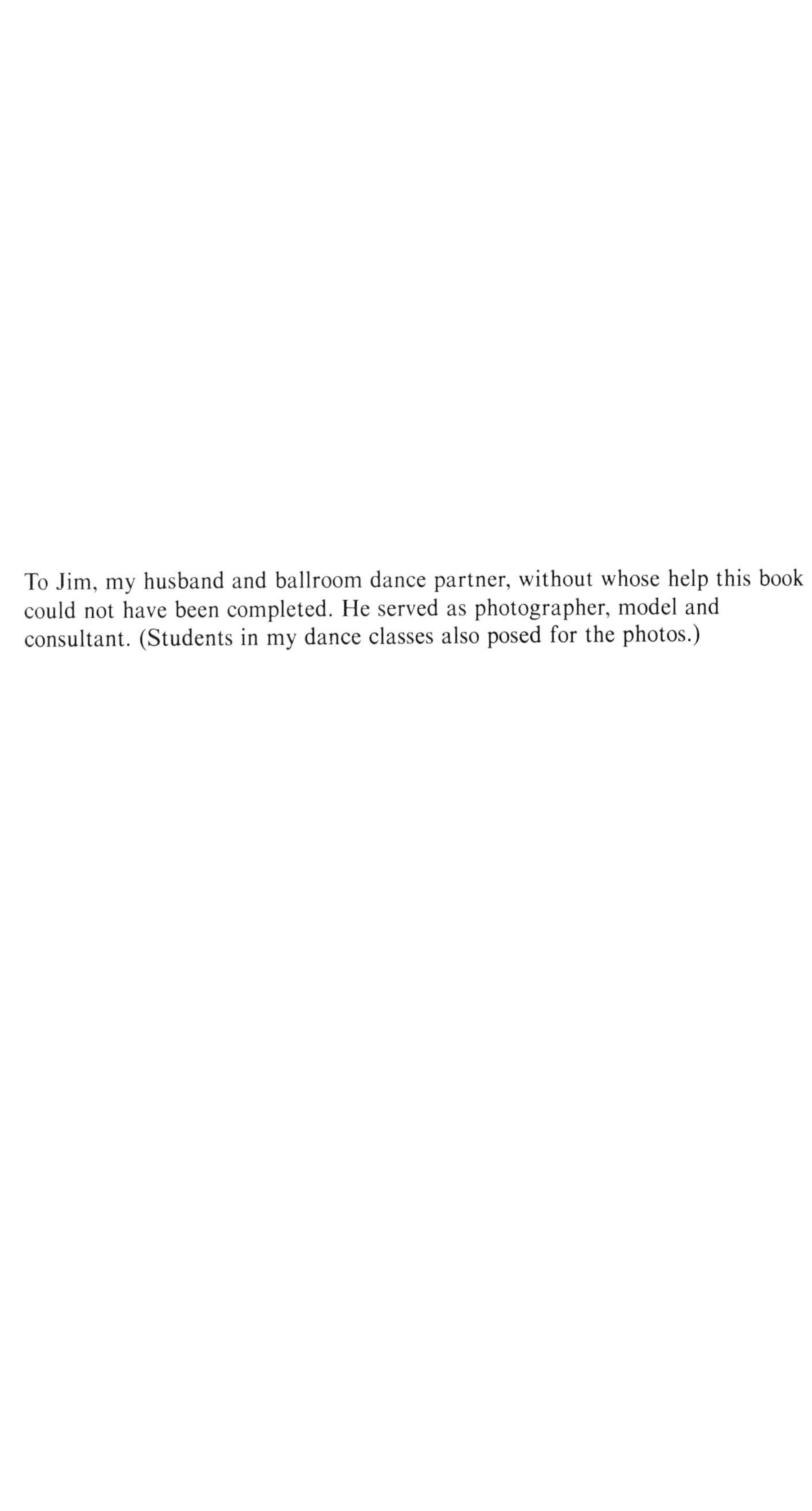

To Jim, my husband and ballroom dance partner, without whose help this book could not have been completed. He served as photographer, model and consultant. (Students in my dance classes also posed for the photos.)

contents

preface

With the advent of the physical fitness boom, dance has flourished. Social dance offers a gregarious approach to healthful exercise. Its aerobic effects range from high-intensity to low-intensity, depending on the skill and energy level of its participants. It emphasizes the elements of balance, rhythm and coordination. It also encourages creative expression and serves as an outlet for the release of stress and tension. As the name implies, the social aspect of social dance is the primary reason for its continuous popularity. It provides opportunities for meeting other active people who share a mutual desire to socialize. The beauty of all these attributes is that social dance is a lifetime recreational activity. It can be compatible with the personal needs of almost any age group.

This book begins with a brief review of the background and development of social dance. It has been said that if one wants to get to know a people and their ways, one should study their dance (Agnes DeMille). Social dance has been influenced by geographical location, social customs and historical facts. The remainder of Chapter 1 is concerned with introducing the novice dancer to the fundamentals of social dance, which will be referred to often throughout the text.

The dances to be learned have been divided into two categories, each of which have defined commonalities. The classification of the smooth dances consists of the fox-trot, waltz and tango. The material is arranged so that the beginner will gradually be introduced to the basics and will be able to interrelate dances and foot patterns within the smooth dance category. These foundations will also carry over to the rhythm dance category, which consists of the remainder of ballroom dances that cannot be classified as smooth dances. This system simplifies the learning process.

The format for each dance usually consists of a brief history, timing, styling, basic step(s), variations and turns. Line drawings, musical measures and photographs are used as aids to the learner. At the end of each chapter, a suggested sequence of steps and suggested musical selections are provided. Record Sources, a list of Social Dance Record Albums, Suggested Teaching Procedures and references in the Bibliography are available in the Appendixes.

The starting position for each dance is the basic closed position unless noted otherwise. Most of the dances and variations are presented in the order of difficulty. Both the man's and the women's parts are described, but the women's part is usually in natural opposition to the man's part. Most of the step patterns are repeated four times when developing sequences. Turning variations are often repeated three times in order to prevent vertigo. It also helps to "spot," which consists of continuous rotation of the head so as to watch a certain spot on the wall. As each new step pattern is added, routines should be gradually developed and practiced. Spontaneous leading and following of these variations is also important. Partners should be changed often. As the students progress, the creative approach, involving innovative variations and routines, should be encouraged as the ultimate in social dance skill and comprehension. An advanced method of dance exhibition on the college level is called formation dancing. It consists of teams of six or eight couples who create designs and step patterns for ballroom-dance competition. For further information, contact the Imperial Society of Teachers of Dancing in London, England, or refer to Record Sources in the Appendixes.

The reader who desires further visual instruction to accompany this text should contact the author for the SOCIAL DANCE video tape. The author's zip code is 62026.

Social
Dance

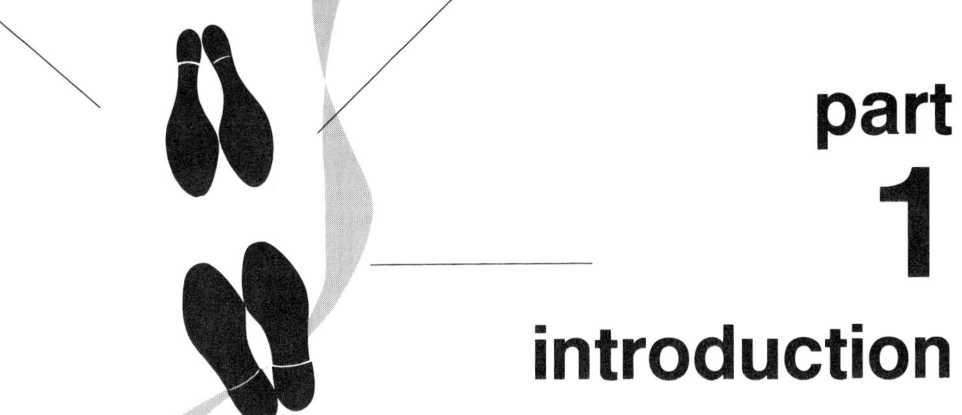

part
1

introduction

background and general information

1

Although dance began as an expression of human movement in primitive times, the presence of social dance was insignificant until the fifteenth century, around the time of the Renaissance in Europe. Here, the aristocrats engaged in refined couple court dances while the peasants enjoyed participating in the less sophisticated, robust and rowdy, traditional folk dances.

In New England in the early 1600s, mixed dancing was forbidden in the American colonies, and participants were punished severely by Puritans. Further south, Virginia was settled by a higher social class of people from England who considered dancing to be an important aspect of proper etiquette. By the end of the 1600s, dancing masters were plentiful. Social dance had become widely accepted by the time of the American Revolution. Balls, country dances, jigs and cotillions were popular forms of dancing in the American's social life.

The next dance craze occurred in the 1830s when both Europe and America embraced the whirling dance steps of the waltz and the polka. At first, these dances were proclaimed "indecent" because they dared to require a closed-couple (face-to-face) dance position. But their popularity was not to be denied, and social dance became the predominant force in recreational activity. Once again, class distinction was evident from the great society balls to the dance hall concert saloons. By the end of the nineteenth century, all class levels were actively involved in social dance, and dance education was gaining acceptance. Soon, the art of social dance was added to the physical education programs of the schools. Also, during the twentieth century, many new forms of social dance were developed.

POPULAR DANCES OF THE TWENTIETH CENTURY

1900s—The cakewalk, the can-can and the one-step were the rage.

1910—The tango was welcomed from the Argentine.

1911—The turkey trot and other animal-named dances arrived.

1913—The fox-trot, enduring in popularity, was introduced.

1917—The castle walk was presented by the famous dancing Castles.

1920s—The Jazz Age produced the shocking shimmy, the black bottom and the Charleston. They symbolized the rebellious attitude characteristic of the times.

1927—The lindy hop (the first of many jitterbug-style dances) was devised in honor of Charles Lindbergh's solo flight across the Atlantic Ocean.

1930—The rumba ("queen" of the Latin dances) was greeted from Cuba.

1930s—The big "swing" bands era began and lasted into the next decade. Huge crowds were packed into dance halls all over the United States.

1940s—The samba was brought from Brazil, and the Cubans supplied the mambo and the cha-cha (or triple mambo). Brief encounters with the big apple and the shag were enjoyed by the younger set.

1950s—The merengue from Haiti intrigued dancers. Rock and roll began its great impact and stressed a jitterbug-swing style of dance. Various specialized fads like the mashed potatoes, the stroll, the twist and others became popular.

1960s—The individualized fad dances and the effects of the Viet Nam War dramatically changed the style of dancing in the United States. Acid rock and discotheque dance emphasized a free style to accompany the loud sounds, bright lights and flashing stobes.

1970s—Disco dance evolved, and couple or "touch" dancing was reinstated.

1980s—Country-swing and modern-style rock again emphasized couple dancing.

FOOT POSITIONS

These five foot positions (fig.1.1) are universal to dance, exercise and attitudizational posing. They were derived from ballet technique, which was developed in 1700, but the degree of turnout approached a straight line or 180 degrees. Most other types of dance incorporate a modified version called the five parallel foot positions. The social dancer will often refer to these basic positions of stance.

POSTURE

Good posture contributes to effective and efficient dance movement, and a dancer must have proper body carriage in order to look proficient. Posture is of utmost importance, especially at the beginning of the learning experience so that bad habits can be prevented. To start, assume the first foot position and stand erect, observing these cues:

1. The body weight is slightly forward on the ball of the foot with the heels barely touching the floor.
2. Bend the knees slightly to be ready for movement.
3. The next step is to contract the lower torso to flatten the abdomen and the waist or lumbar region of the back.

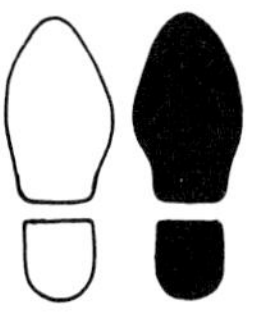

a. First position

a. Feet are slightly apart (one or two inches) and toes point straight ahead on a straight line.

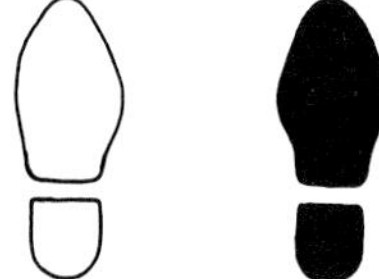

b. Second position

b. Feet are shoulder width apart with toes pointing straight ahead and on a straight line. Weight is evenly distributed on both feet. Second position is equivalent to side-stride position.

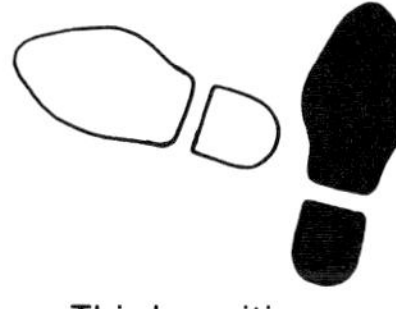

c. Third position

c. Cue: Heel to instep. One foot points straight ahead, the other is perpendicular at the instep. Note: in the parallel version, the toes point straight ahead with one foot slightly advanced one-half foot length.

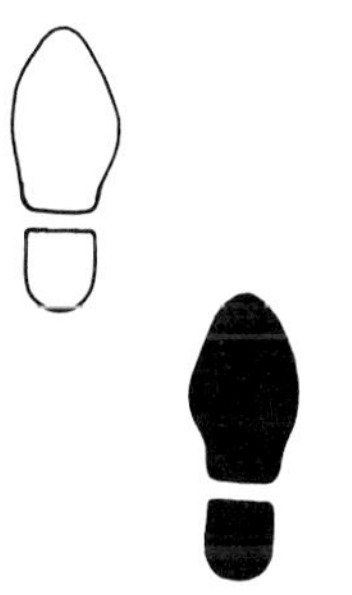

d. Fourth position

d. Both feet point straight ahead, but the leading foot is 12 to 18 inches forward of the rear foot. Fourth position is equivalent to forward stride position. Weight is equally distributed on both feet.

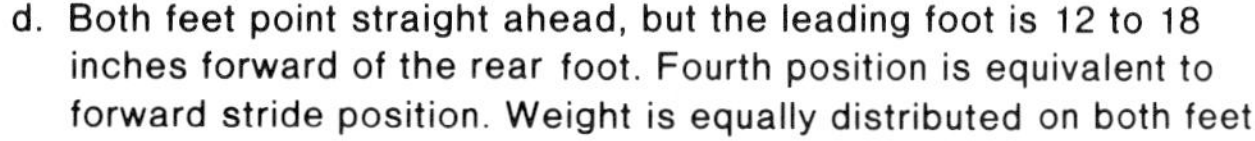

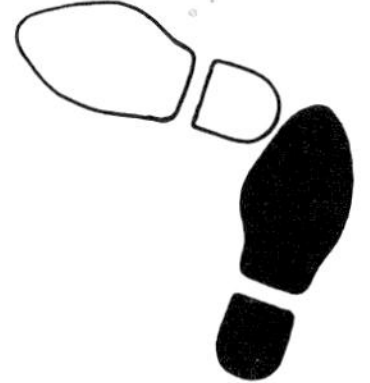

e. Fifth position

e. Cue: Heel to toe. One foot points straight ahead, the other is perpendicular at the toes. Note: in the parallel version, the toes point straight ahead with one foot advanced one full foot length. Also, crossed feet are indicative of fifth position.

Figure 1.1. Foot positions

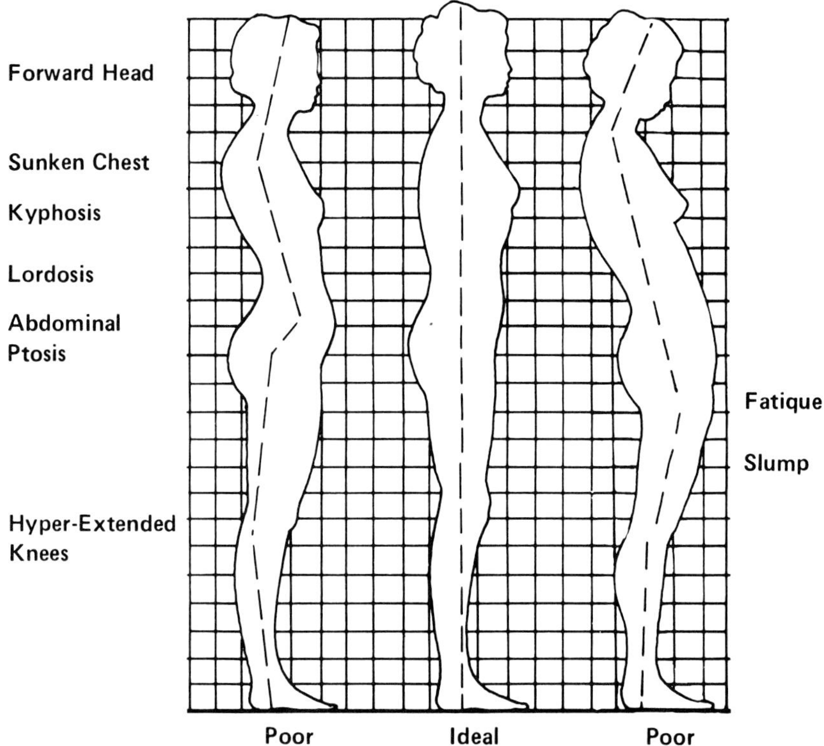

Figure 1.2. Body alignment (From Lindsey, Jones, Whitley, FITNESS, Wm. C. Brown Company Pubishers, 1983, p. 88.)

4. Separate the upper and lower torso by lifting the midriff and then the chest.
5. Shoulders back and flatten the scapulae or shoulder blades.
6. The head is erect with the chin down and in, and the back of the head is up.

If the body is properly aligned, a side-view plumb line will bisect these points: mid-earlobe, mid-shoulder, mid-hip, and slightly forward of the mid-knee and mid-ankle bone. If the line does not bisect these points, postural deviations can be detected.

1. Forward head—the mid-earlobe is forward of the plumb line.
2. Sunken chest—flat chest.
3. Kyphosis—(round upper back) the shoulder blades protrude.
4. Stooped shoulders—the tip of the shoulder is forward.
5. Lordosis—(sway or hollow back) the hips are forward of the line, and there is an increased lumbar curve.
6. Abdominal ptosis—(protruding abdomen) abdominal muscles sag.
7. Hyperextended knees—knees are too straight (locked).

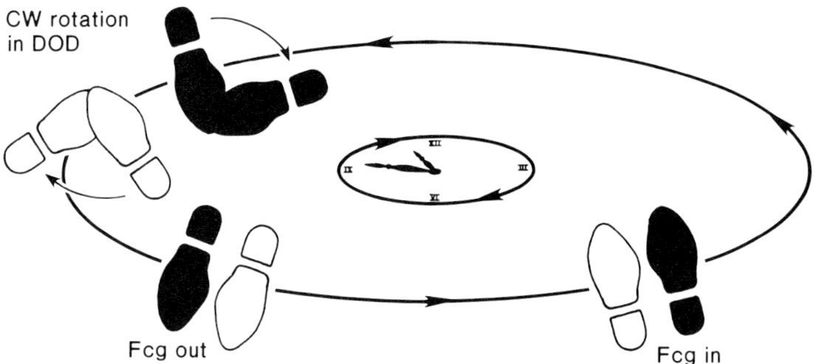

Figure 1.3. Direction of dance

8. Fatigue slump—all of these deviations are evident. Specifically prescribed exercises that are performed on a regular basis will correct these functional deviations. The structural deviations, which are not included here, are more serious and usually cannot be corrected through exercise.

Find someone to check your best standing posture from a side view. Determine whether there are deviations to be corrected. Try altering the position of alignment to correct minor deviations. Determine which muscles need to be strengthened in order to hold the framework and soft parts of the body in position.

DIRECTION OF DANCE

This is also known as *line of direction* or *line of dance*. It refers to the direction of travel on the dance floor. Envision the route as a highway; the dancers avoid collisions if they adhere to the rules of the road. They progress in a counter-clockwise direction or opposite to the movement of the hands on a clock.

DIRECTIONS OF MOVEMENT

The novice dancer needs to learn to move in various directions. Initially, each dancer should face direction of dance or counter-clockwise and assume a well-aligned position of proper standing posture. The arms could be held sideward to form a "W" (hence, the name "W-position") to serve as a preliminary to the basic couple dance position. The lone dancer should attempt to move confidently in all directions. To accomplish this, first swing the indicated leg forward and backward from the knee for a limited range of motion. Swing the leg from the hip for a comparison of the increased range of motion. Then reach forward, from the hip, stepping onto the heel first as in a normal walk. (Some instructors prefer to teach stepping onto the toes first as in the ballet walk.) Continue walking forward, allowing two counts for each step. This is designated as "slow." The toes should point almost straight ahead. (Some instructors prefer to teach that the

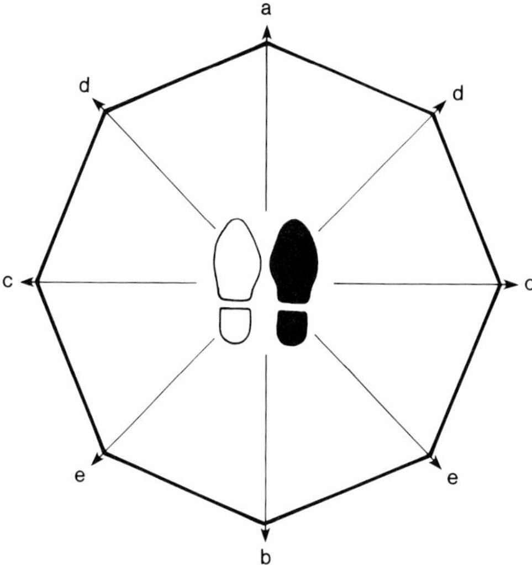

a. L or R foot forward
b. L or R foot backward
c. L or R foot sideward
d. L or R foot diagonally forward
e. L or R foot diagonally backward

Figure 1.4. Directions of movement

toes point slightly outward as in the ballet walk.) Pass the feet closely so that the knees almost brush, but keep the weight centered though slightly on the outer borders of the feet. Lift the foot slightly off the floor to avoid the appearance of dragging the feet. Transfer the weight smoothly and maintain balance.

To reverse the direction, reach backward from the hip, stepping onto the toes first as in a normal backward walk. Otherwise, the same cues apply.

To step sideward, the working foot is placed about twelve inches from the other foot to the designated side and takes the weight. The other foot is then closed adjacent to it. For a smooth transference of weight, push slightly with the supporting foot first before stepping with the working foot. One count or "quick" is alloted for each step. The cue of "side-together" can be given and/or "quick, quick."

Try also stepping in diagonals to complete the exercise. See figure 1.4.

BASIC CLOSED-COUPLE DANCE POSITION

This is also known as *social dance position.* The couple faces foresquare in good standing posture.

The man's part:

1. He faces direction of dance.

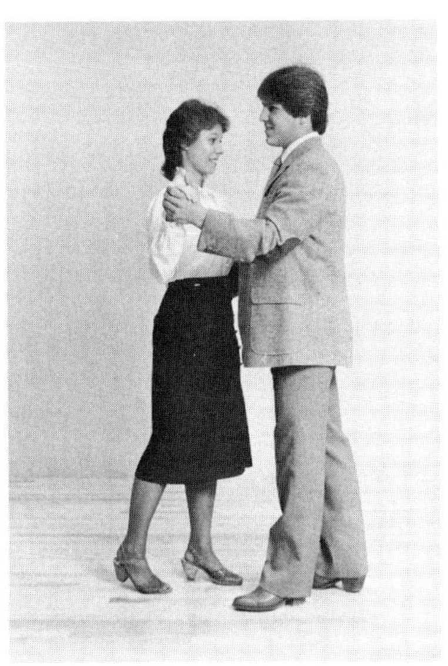

Figure 1.5. Closed position

2. His left arm is extended toward the center of the counter-clockwise circle. The palm of his left hand faces forward, with the elbow bent and slightly lower than the shoulder.
3. His right arm slopes downward, and the hand, with fingers together and palm cupped, is placed below the woman's left shoulder blade near the spine.
4. He looks over the woman's right shoulder.

The woman's part:

1. She faces her partner directly, looking over his right shoulder. Her feet are a few inches forward of his.
2. Her right arm is extended toward the center of the circle, with her hand facing forward and her fingers placed between the man's thumb and forefinger of his left hand.
3. She supports the weight of her left arm, which rests lightly on the man's upper right arm. Their elbows meet, even if the couple's heights are not compatible, and her left hand with fingers together should continue its direction toward the point of the man's right shoulder.

This basic closed couple dance position will vary with the specific style and form of each dance. These changes will be made later as different dances are studied. The basic position described will apply to the fox-trot and the waltz, and it will be modified for the tango by a slight exaggeration of the elevation of the arms.

OTHER IMPORTANT SOCIAL DANCE POSITIONS

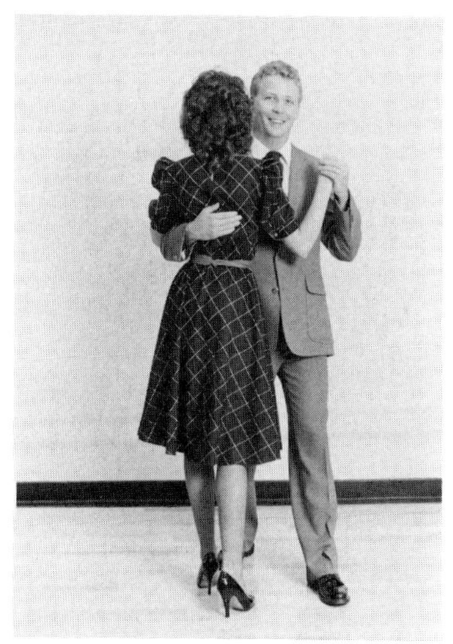

Figure 1.6. Right parallel position

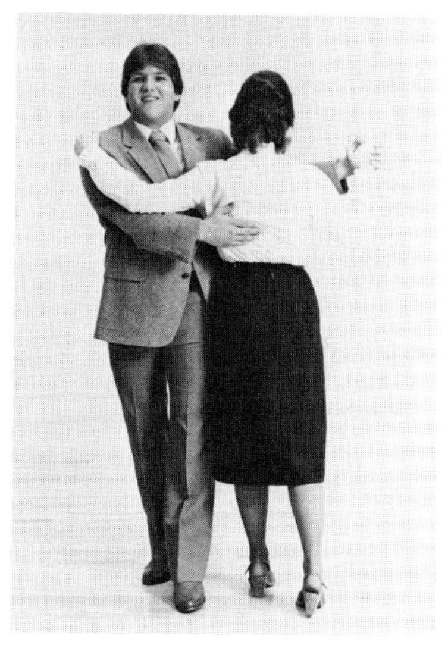

Figure 1.7. Left parallel position

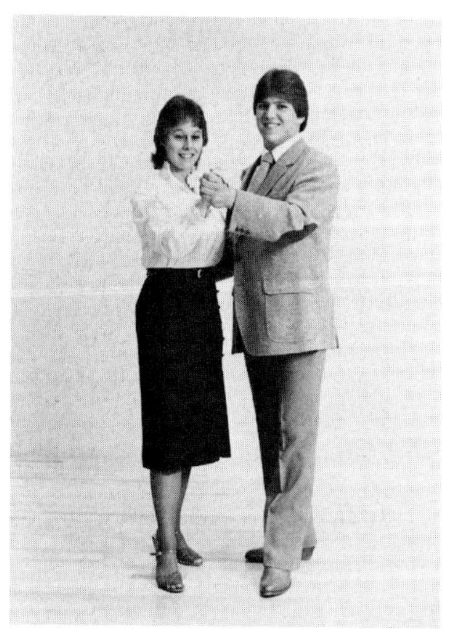

Figure 1.8. Conversation position

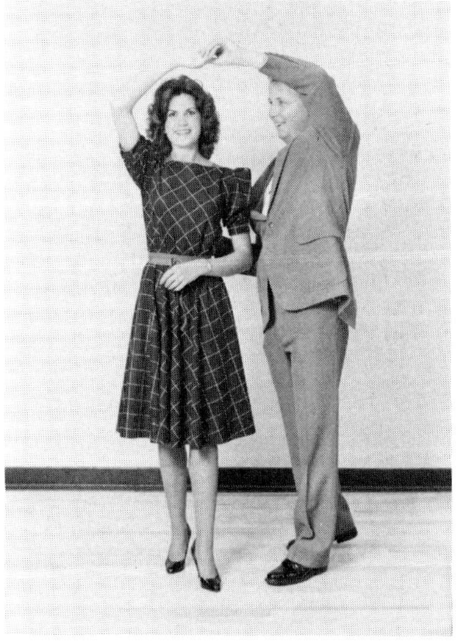

Figure 1.9. Arch position

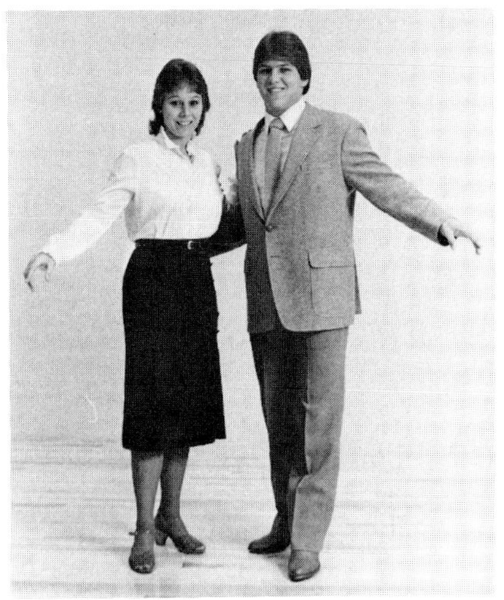

a

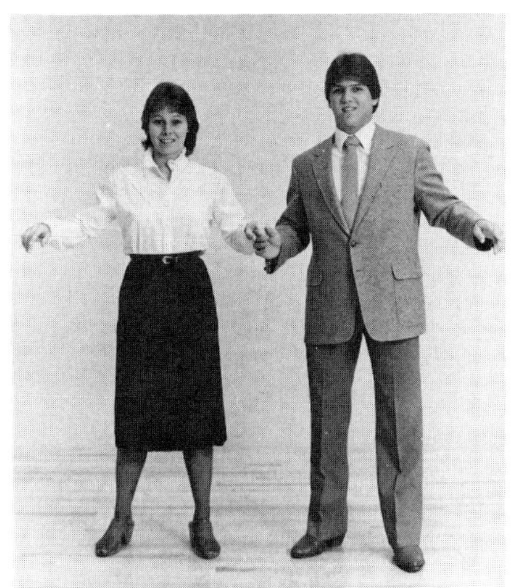

b

Figure 1.10. *a,* Open position; *b,* full open position

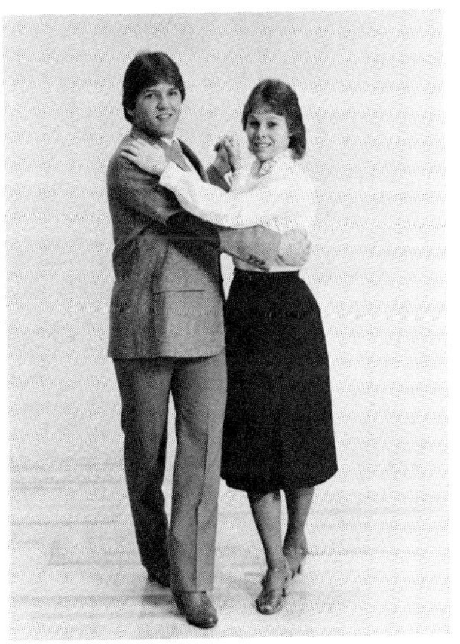

Figure 1.11. Reverse position

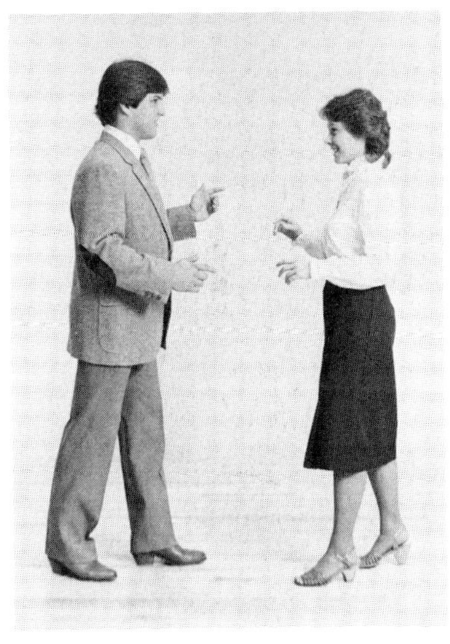

Figure 1.12. Shine position

LEADING AND FOLLOWING

Leading

On the dance floor, the man is expected to take an assertive role as the leader. (In accordance with modern role changes, the woman might occasionally attempt to be the assertive party if circumstances permit.) He is responsible for the choice of steps, direction, rhythm and pace. To develop this skill, the man must know the steps. This is essential in leading. After learning the step patterns well, he must also learn to convey his intentions to his partner so they can move together in a compatible manner.

The requirements of good leading consist of firm control and proper body position. The man will probably be instructed to move his upper torso and right hand momentarily before moving his feet, but when viewing this process, the body parts appear to move simultaneously. As he steps forward, he also indicates the forward direction of movement with a slight pressure of his left hand. As he steps backward, he uses pressure with the palm of his right hand. A sideward lead consists of a slight nudge in the intended direction. To turn the woman to her right, the man uses the heel of his right hand. To turn the woman to her left, he uses the fingers of his right hand. The man should determine the proper leads for each step pattern and time them for smooth execution. Be sure to finish the previous step pattern before changing the leads for another.

Cues

1. As the music begins to play, listen to the timing (not the melody), decide which dance is appropriate and mentally envision definite step patterns.
2. The man usually starts forward with his left foot on count one.
3. Begin with simple, well-executed basic steps and gradually increase the difficulty as the dancers progress together. The same step should be performed at least twice and usually four times in succession. The transition from one step pattern to another should be fluid and smooth. The leader's skill is tested especially when dancing with a new partner for the first time.
4. Verbalization of leads is unnecessary and often annoying.
5. If either partner loses time with the music, they should complete the present step pattern, pause to listen to the beat and then attempt to regain the proper tempo.
6. The leader should try to enhance the appearance of his partner so that their shared experience is pleasant and enjoyed by both dancers.
7. Look straight ahead, not down at the feet.
8. Practice. Changing partners often is very effective.

Following

Although the woman is delegated the more passive role in social dance, she has certain responsibilities in the partnership. She is expected to:

1. know the step-patterns and some of the variations;
2. offer responsive resistance;

3. avoid foot collisions by taking longer strides;
4. maintain dynamic posture so that movement can be made in any direction;
5. be aware of the man's possible lead indications;
6. obtain better balance by placing the left hand firmly near the back of the man's right shoulder;
7. initially be ready to step backward with the right foot; and
8. practice (she might even try to lead another woman so as to gain a better understanding of both parts).

ETIQUETTE

The word etiquette is an old-fashioned term, but its significance in social affairs should not be regarded as antiquated. It envelops a sense of respect for the feelings of other people and basic rules concerning good manners, which are rarely altered.

Whether in dance class or at a social affair, the appropriate way to ask for a dance is: "May I have this dance?" If accepted, the intended should be escorted to and from the dance floor. If rejected, consent should not be immediately given to another. While on the dance floor, these offensive actions are considered to be rude, discourteous and impolite: showing off or "hogging" the floor, constant chattering, stonefaced silence, insistent instruction while dancing, resisting the general flow of traffic and other forms of impudent behavior. The custom of "cutting in" on another couple is usually accepted in the United States unless the scene is a public place involving strangers. Other countries often find this practice questionable. In dance class, "cutting in" can be a useful tool and an enjoyable experience when dealing with extras who have no partner. As a final gesture, the partners should thank each other for the dance(s). The rules of etiquette involve good common sense when dealing with other people and insure that all who wish to socialize will have a good time.

RHYTHMIC AWARENESS

If the novice has had little previous experience in dance or music, moving to the beat of the music should be emphasized. The instruments usually responsible for carrying the underlying beat are the drums, bass and piano. The Latin rhythms incorporate the clavs (sticks), bongo drums and wood block. Beginners should first be taught the correct way to clap the hands or tap the feet to the underlying beat of the music and then should attempt to participate. When this is mastered, they should try to step out on every beat and then only on the accented beats which are counts one and three in four-count music and count one in three-count music. The slow rhythms require a long, slow step, and the fast rhythms require a short, fast step. When the students are ready, partners should be added so as to progress toward performing the steps together in time with the music. The teacher will be responsible for giving verbal cues such as the length of the musical introduction, the correct rhythm for phrases and changes and when to start.

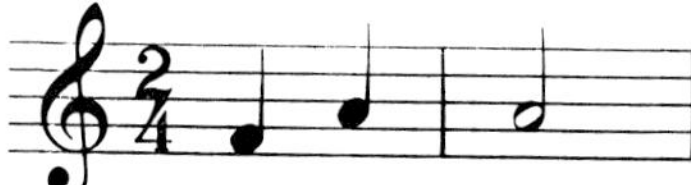

Figure 1.13. Measure

Rhythm is motion through time. The beat measures time through regular pulses. Some beats are stressed or accented to become stronger than others. A measure is a group of regularly occurring strong and weak beats and is enclosed between two adjacent bars on a musical staff. The meter refers to the grouping of beats into a musical pattern. The time signature is a symbol of the metric pattern of each measure, such as $\frac{2}{4}$; the top number indicates that there are two beats in a measure, and the bottom number signifies that a quarter note receives one beat. Other common time signatures in social dance are $\frac{4}{4}$, $\frac{6}{4}$ and $\frac{6}{8}$. The waltz is designated $\frac{3}{4}$ most commonly, but it could in some instances be $\frac{3}{8}$, $\frac{3}{2}$ or $\frac{9}{8}$. When the bottom number is an eight, an eighth note receives one beat; a two signifies that a half note receives one beat.

ABBREVIATIONS

A list of abbreviations has been compiled as an aid in the description of step patterns throughout the text.

Bwd	Backward		Mnvr	Manuever
Bsd	Beside		Opp	Opposite
CCW	Counter-clockwise		Orig	Original
Chg	Change		Pos	Position
Ct	Count		q	Quick
Ctr	Center		R	Right
CW	Clockwise		S	Slow
Diag	Diagonal		Sd	Side
Dir	Direction		Sl	Slightly
Dr	Draw		Str	Straight
Fcg	Facing		Tch	Touch
Frt	Front		Tog	Together
Ft	Foot		Twd	Toward
Fwd	Forward		Thru	Through
Ho	Hold		Var	Variation
IP	In Place		Wt	Weight
L	Left		X	Cross

INTERPRETING THE DIAGRAMS

Dotted line with an arrow --→ The path of the left foot is traced.

Solid line with an arrow ——→ The path of the right foot is traced.

Half foot — The foot is touched to the floor (no weight change).

Whole foot — Weight change takes place.

White foot — Left foot placement

Black foot — Right foot placement

Man   Woman

Cues:

1. Locate "start."
2. Find ct 1 (L white ft for man, R black ft for woman) and proceed to other consecutive cts in S's and q's.
3. Determine dir (lines and arrows) and placement of each ft.
4. Practice.

Note: The woman's foot patterns will usually face the opposite direction so as to assimilate her dance position in relation to the man. Her illustrations must be rotated 180 degrees to visualize and practice her part.

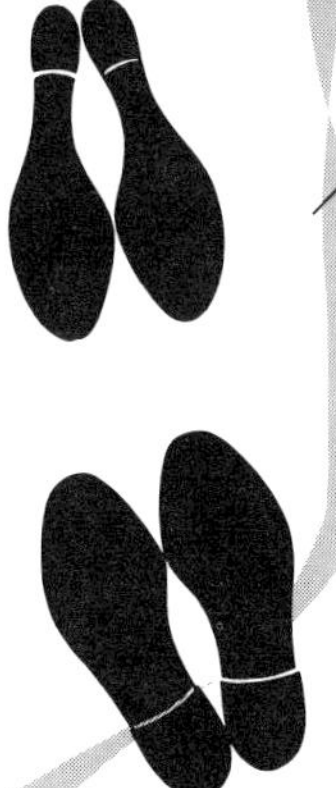

part
2

smooth dances

The smooth dances include the fox-trot, the waltz and the tango. The dance fundamentals introduced in Part 1 provide a solid basis for our continuation of social dance technique. Again emphasize erect posture with the arms and shoulders elevated in the closed-couple dance position and long, gliding steps originating from the hip. Eventually, as the dancers progress, other common characteristics of smooth dancing can be considered. These include the ultimate in advanced leading skill, which incorporates close body contact at the diaphragm area of the torso and advanced follow-through technique at the end of each continuous step pattern to produce a fluid, uninterrupted series of steps.

The smooth dances, sometimes referred to as "slow dancing," should be a vision of graceful movement with limited jerking or jiggering. The streamlined steps should blend together effortlessly with no apparent strain or fatigue. Relax and enjoy!

Peanuts

featuring

"Good ol' Charlie Brown"

by Schulz

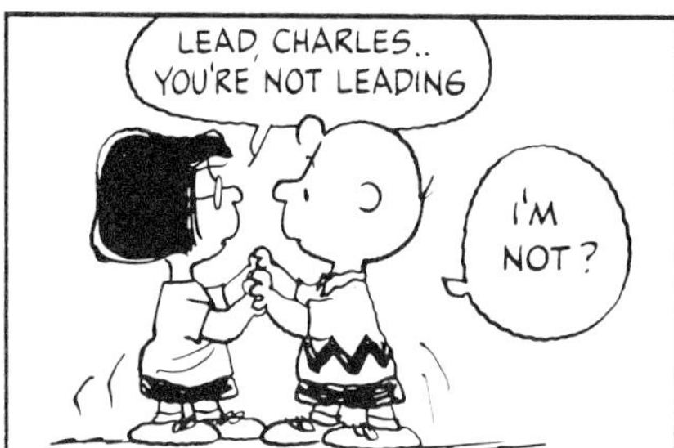

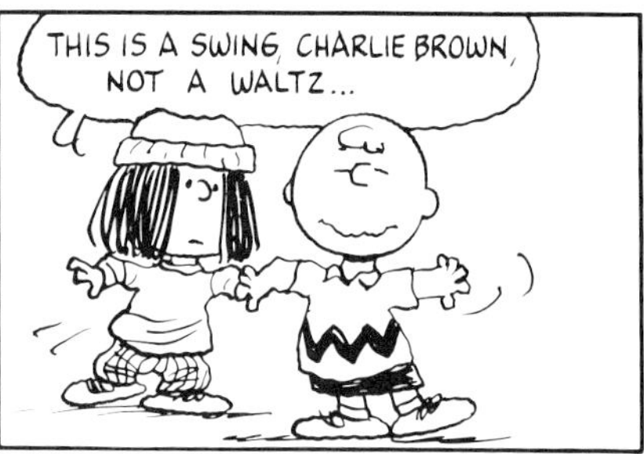

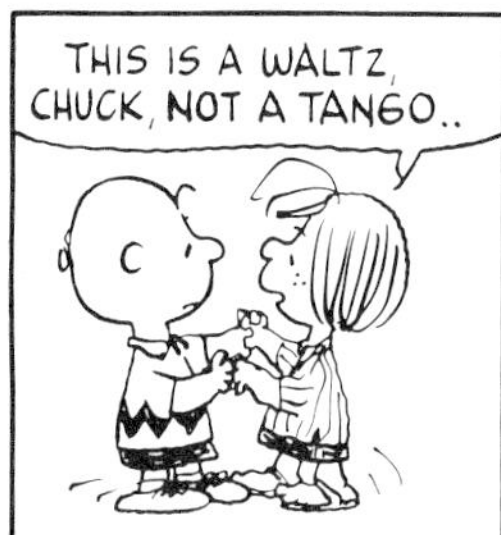

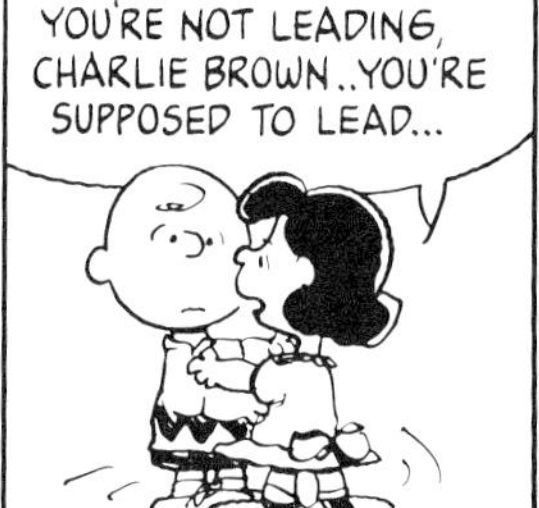

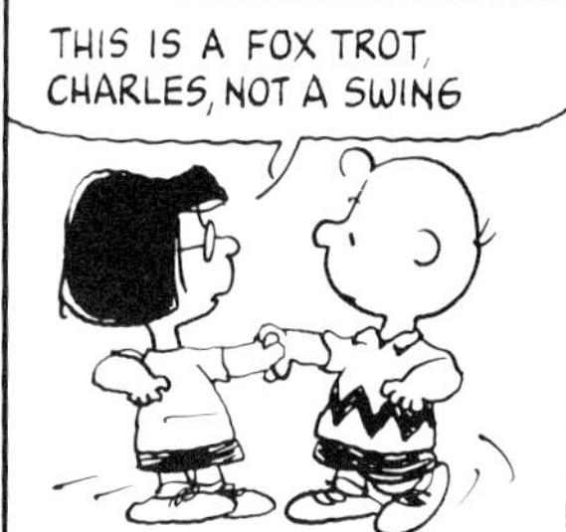

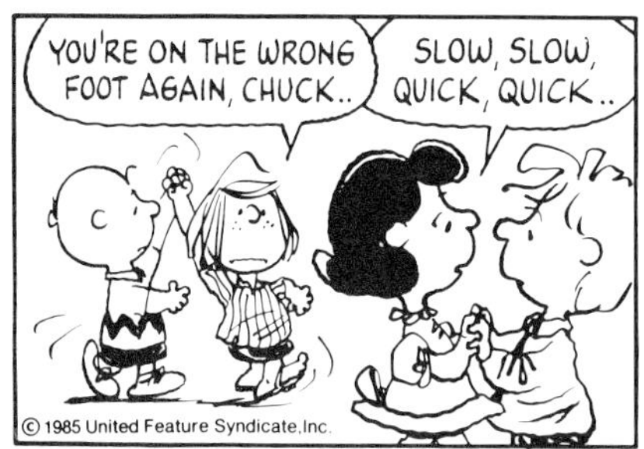

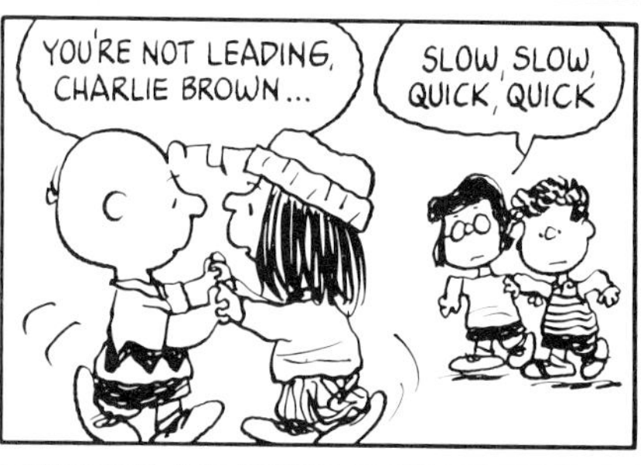

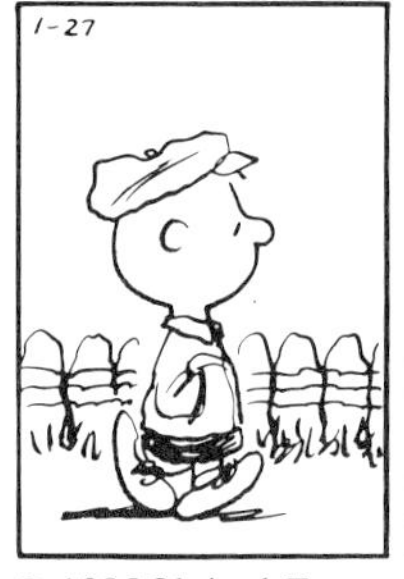

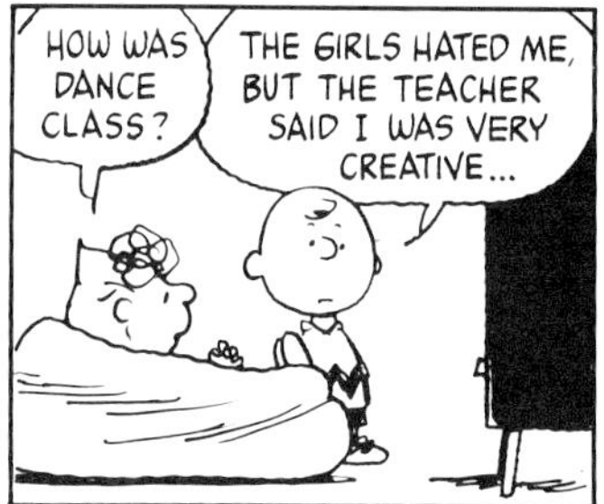

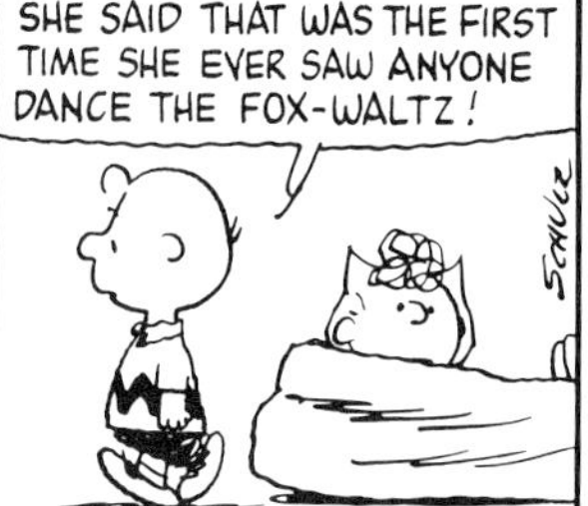

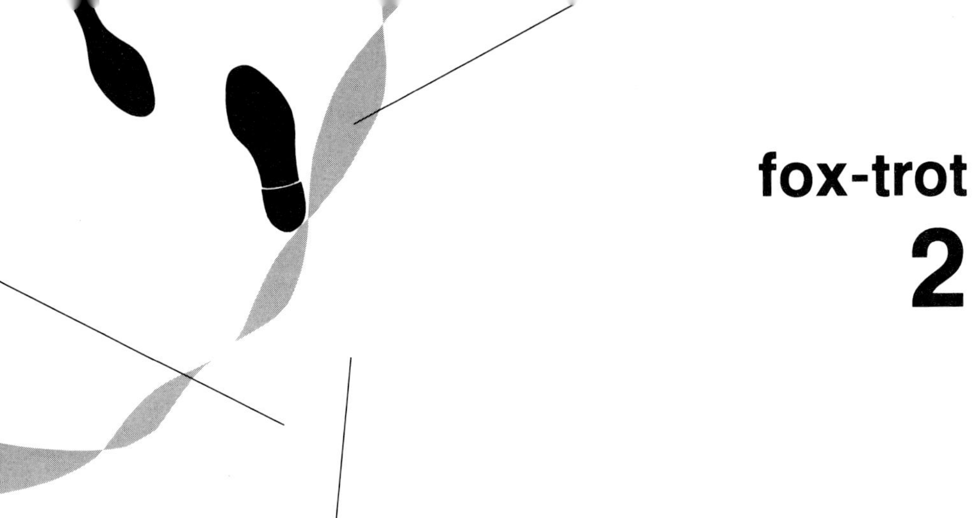

fox-trot

2

In 1913, Harry Fox performed a continuous trotting step in his popular vaudeville act and became the founder of the only truly American ballroom dance. This pristine version developed into a one-step (all quicks) and a two-step (three quicks in the count of two) to be compatible with the lively ragtime and jazz rhythms. Though the $\frac{2}{4}$ renditions endured, a slower $\frac{4}{4}$ variation was also devised to include four slow walking steps and eight quick running steps. Professional dancers like Vernon and Irene Castle embraced the fox-trot rhythms and developed the smooth style which is characteristic of the dance. New patterns like the box step evolved, and later, Arthur Murray invented the magic step basic which could be used in 27 different ways. Throughout the eras of swing, rock and roll, disco, country, rock and others, fox-trot has survived in various forms to become America's all-time favorite dance.

Timing

The fox-trot tempo may vary from fast to slow, but the beginner will prefer slow music at first. The time signature should be $\frac{4}{4}$ with counts one and three heavily accented. A basic step pattern with the rhythm of slow, quick, quick will require one measure of music, and a slow, slow, quick, quick pattern will require one and a half measures of music.

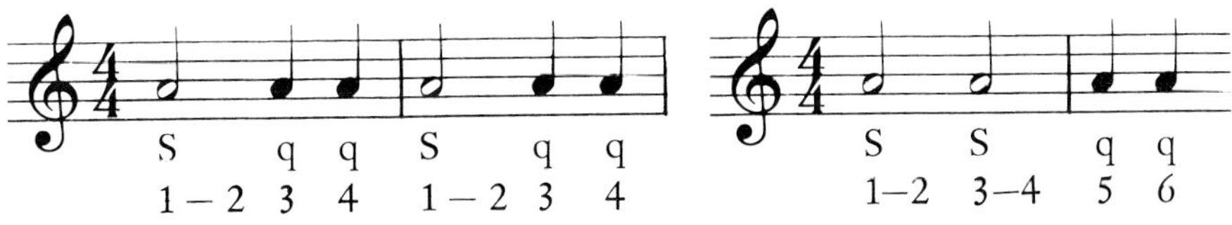

Figure 2.1.

Styling

The fox-trot is a traveling dance; its basic component is the most elementary form of locomotion, the walk. It has been said that if you can walk, you can dance. This is true, especially in fox-trot. Whether the walk is performed forward, backward or sideward, natural form and graceful body line should be emphasized. The term smooth dances has been derived from their smooth style, and the fox-trot has been instrumental in this conception.

Basic Steps

The two step patterns considered to be basic to fox-trot are the box step and Arthur Murray's magic step. The primary difference in the two is the number of slow steps required. The box step has one slow step and the magic step has two slow steps. (The starting position will be the basic closed-couple dance position unless otherwise specified.) When a change of direction is imminent, the unweighted foot will touch beside the weighted foot for one count; otherwise, the free foot follows through.

The Box Step

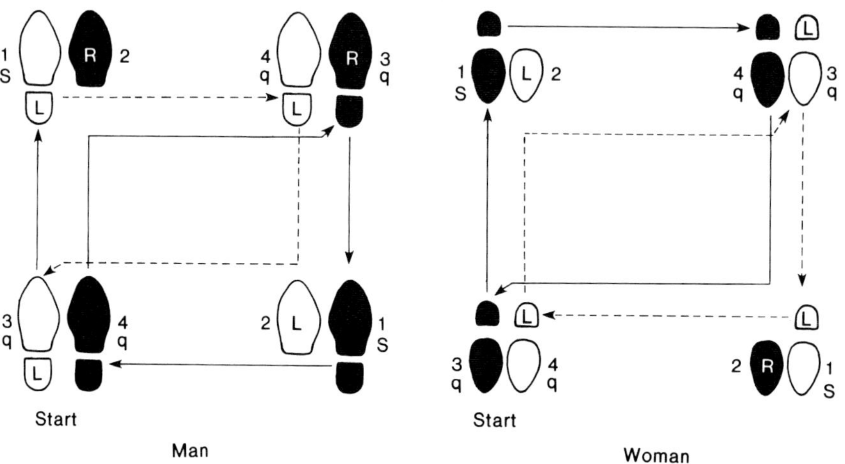

Figure 2.2. Box step

Step	Foot	Directional Cue	Count	Timing Cue	Comments
Forward Half Box					
1	Lt	Fwd	1–2	S	On ct 2, touch R ft beside L ft (no wt chg) in 1st pos. of ft.
2	Rt	Rt sd	3	q	2nd pos. of ft.
3	Lt	Tog	4	q	1st pos. of ft.

Step	Foot	Directional Cue	Count	Timing Cue	Comments
Backward Half Box					
1	Rt	Bwd	1–2	S	On ct 2, touch R ft beside L ft (no wt chg) in 1st pos. of ft.
2	Lt	Lt sd	3	q	2nd pos. of ft.
3	Rt	Tog	4	q	1st pos. of ft.

Note: The man's and woman's parts are in natural opposition. The man begins with the forward half box while the woman begins with the backward half box. The parts are then alternated to complete the full box step.

The Magic Step

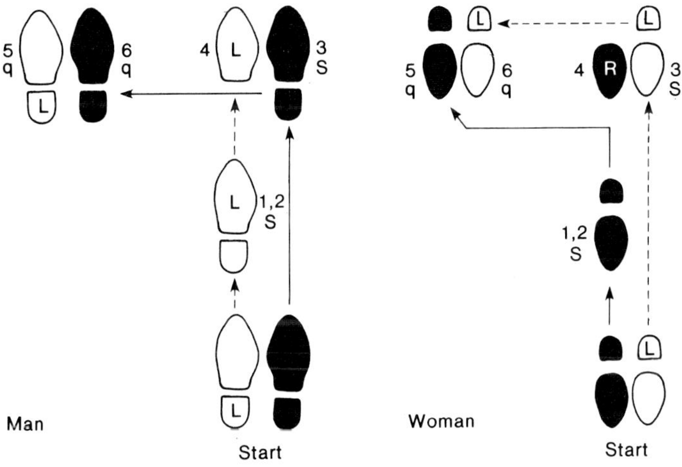

Figure 2.3. Forward magic step

Step	Foot	Directional Cue	Count	Timing Cue	Comments
Forward Magic Step (Man's part)					
1	L	Fwd	1–2	S	cts. 1 & 3 alternate 4th pos.
2	R	Fwd	3–4	S	On ct 4, touch L ft beside R ft (no wt chg) in 1st pos.
3	L	L sd	5	q	2nd pos.
4	R	Tog	6	q	1st pos.

Step	Foot	Directional Cue	Count	Timing Cue	Comments
Woman's Part					
1	R	Bwd	1–2	S	
2	L	Bwd	3–4	S	On ct 4, tch R ft bsd L ft (no wt chg)
3	R	R sd	5	q	
4	L	Tog	6	q	
Backward Magic Step (Man's part)					
1	L	Bwd	1–2	S	
2	R	Bwd	3–4	S	On ct 4, tch L ft bsd R ft (chg of dir imminent)
3	L	Sd	5	q	
4	R	Tog	6	q	
Woman's Part					
1	R	Fwd	1–2	S	
2	L	Fwd	3–4	S	On ct 4, tch R ft bsd L ft (chg of dir. imminent)
3	R	Sd	5	q	
4	L	Tog	6	q	

Variations—Magic Rhythm

Swing Step

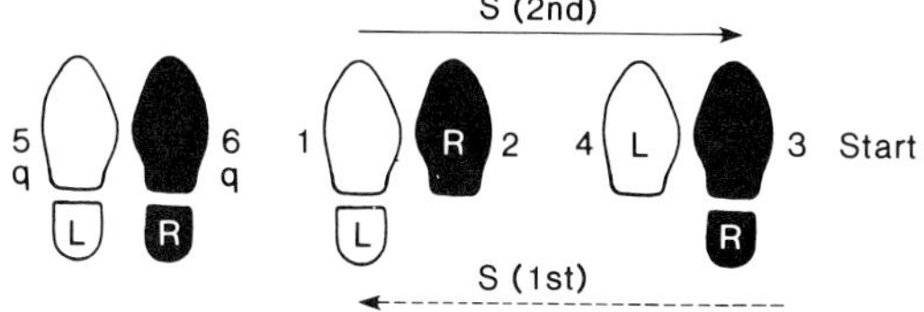

Figure 2.4a. Swing step, man

Step	Foot	Directional Cue	Count	Timing Cue	Comments
Man's Part					
1	L	Sd	1–2	S	On ct 2, tch R ft beside L ft (no wt chg)
2	R	Sd	3–4	S	On ct 4, tch L ft beside R ft (no wt chg)
3	L	Sd	5	q	
4	R	Tog	6	q	

Note: The woman's part is the natural opposite, starting with her R ft to the R sd. The dancers simply move from side to side using magic timing.

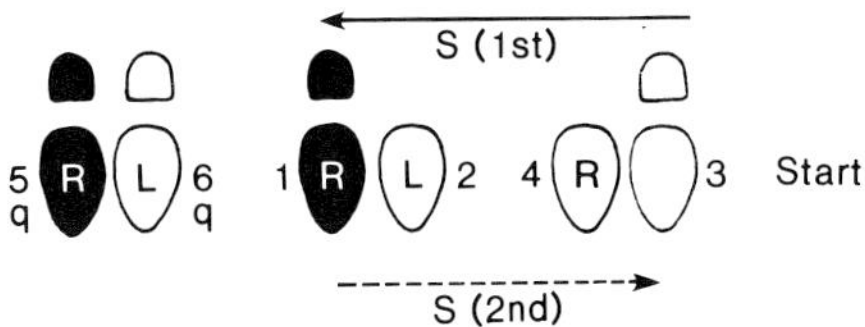

Figure 2.4b. Swing step, woman

Step	Foot	Directional Cue	Count	Timing Cue	Comments
Woman's Part					
1	R	Sd	1–2	S	On ct 2, tch L ft beside R ft (no wt chg)
2	L	Sd	3–4	S	On ct 4, tch R ft beside L ft (no wt chg)
3	R	Sd	5	q	
4	L	Tog	6	q	

Dip or Corte

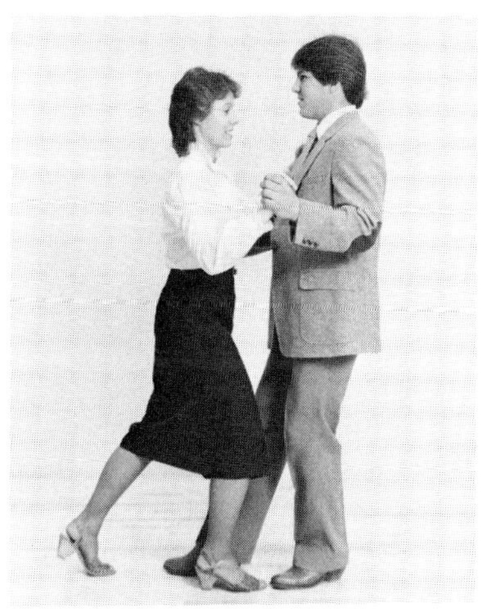

Figure 2.5. Dip

Step	Foot	Directional Cue	Count	Timing Cue	Comments
Man's Part					
1	L	Bwd	1–2	S	Hold backward lunge (4th pos.) on ct 2
2	R	Wt chg Fwd	3–4	S	Recover straight position, ct 4 touch L ft
3	L	Sd	5	q	
4	R	Tog	6	q	

Step	Foot	Directional Cue	Count	Timing Cue	Comments

Note: The dip could be performed in reverse or to the man's L side instead of backward. His L knee must be flexed and over the instep and the R leg is straight. Torso remains erect throughout. The woman's part is the natural opposite (R knee bent, L straight).

Woman's Part

Step	Foot	Directional Cue	Count	Timing Cue	Comments
1	R	Fwd	1–2	S	Hold forward lunge (4th pos.) on ct 2
2	L	Wt chg Bwd	3–4	S	Recover straight pos., ct 4 tch R ft bsd L ft
3	R	Sd	5	q	
4	L	Tog	6	q	

Conversation Step

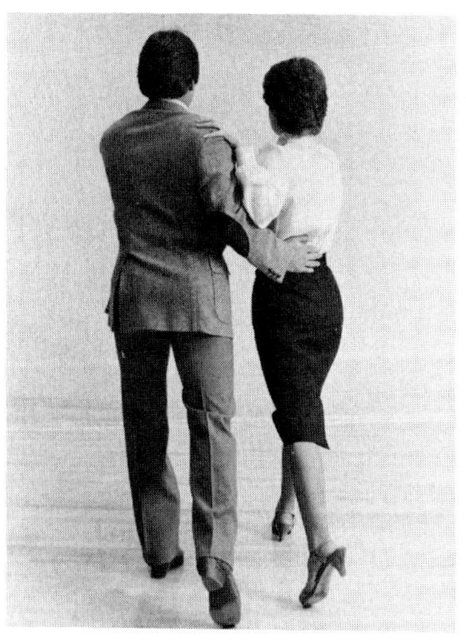

Figure 2.6. Conversation step

Step	Foot	Directional Cue	Count	Timing Cue	Comments
Man's Part					
1	L	Fwd	1–2	S	On ct 1, assume conversation position
2	R	Fwd	3–4	S	Ct 3, R ft follows thru Ct 4, L ft touches beside R and returns to basic closed pos.
3	L	Sd	5	q	(Facing partner)
4	R	Tog	6	q	

Step	Foot	Directional Cue	Count	Timing Cue	Comments

Note: The man's lead for the conversation position is to turn the woman ¼ to her R by opening his rt palm ¼ turn and facing to his L. The couple is then facing the same direction, side by side. Otherwise, the woman's footwork is in natural opposition. The traveling portion of the step pattern should be done in direction of dance. To start, the man faces the outside of the circle, and the woman faces the center of the circle formation. After a method of turning is learned (next section), maneuvers should be made to allow inclusion of the conversation step in sequences. (The cross variation of the magic left turn would be an excellent lead into the conversation step.)

Woman's Part

Step	Foot	Directional Cue	Count	Timing Cue	Comments
1	R	Fwd	1–2	S	On ct 1, assume conversation pos.
2	L	Fwd	3–4	S	Ct 3, L ft follows through Ct 4, R ft tchs bsd L and body assumes basic closed pos.
3	R	Sd	5	q	(facing partner)
4	L	Tog	6	q	

Turns

Magic Left Turn (Magic Rhythm)

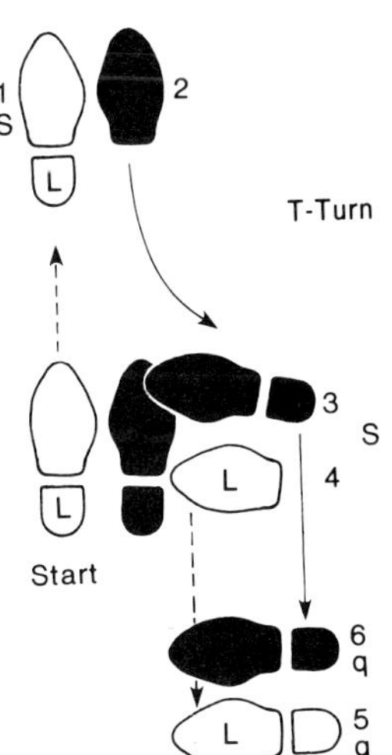

Figure 2.7a. Magic left turn, man

Step	Foot	Directional Cue	Count	Timing Cue	Comments
Man's Part					
1	L	Fwd	1–2	S	Short step, touch R ft beside L ft
2	R	Bwd	3–4	S	Turn R ft ¼ CCW first. Make a "T" with ft. Ct 4 tch L ft beside R
3	L	Sd	5	q	Directly to the L sd
4	R	Tog	6	q	

Note: Keep shoulders square; do not lower L arm during turn. Man uses fingertips of both hands to lead the turn. The woman's part is in natural opposition. On the ¼ turn, the forward L step is arc-shaped with the toe leading. The magic left turn can be a useful tool when a different direction is required.

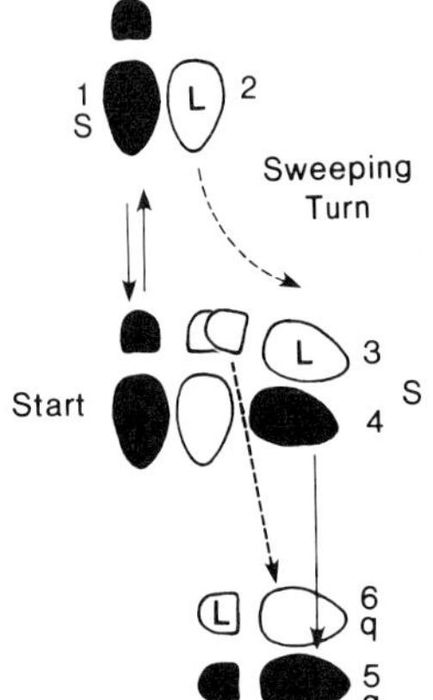

Figure 2.7b. Magic left turn, woman

Step	Foot	Directional Cue	Count	Timing Cue	Comments
Woman's Part					
1	R	Bwd	1–2	S	Short step, tch L ft bsd R ft
2	L	Fwd	3–4	S	Turn L ft ¼ CCW first. "Sweeping" foot fwd. Ct 4 tch L ft bsd R
3	R	Sd	5	q	Step directly to R sd.
4	L	Tog	6	q	

Variations

The magic left turn can be modified by changing only the quicks.

Parallel (R) variation: assume R parallel position on steps 3 and 4. The man uses his fingertips of both hands to lead into this position and the heel of the R hand to lead out of it.

Cross variation: only step 4 (the last quick) is changed. Both the man and woman step through (man's R, woman's L ft) to conversation position. The man leads this with the heel of the R hd.

Left Box Turn (Box Rhythm)

Review the basic box step first. This method of changing direction while using the box step will be very useful as we proceed to other dances.

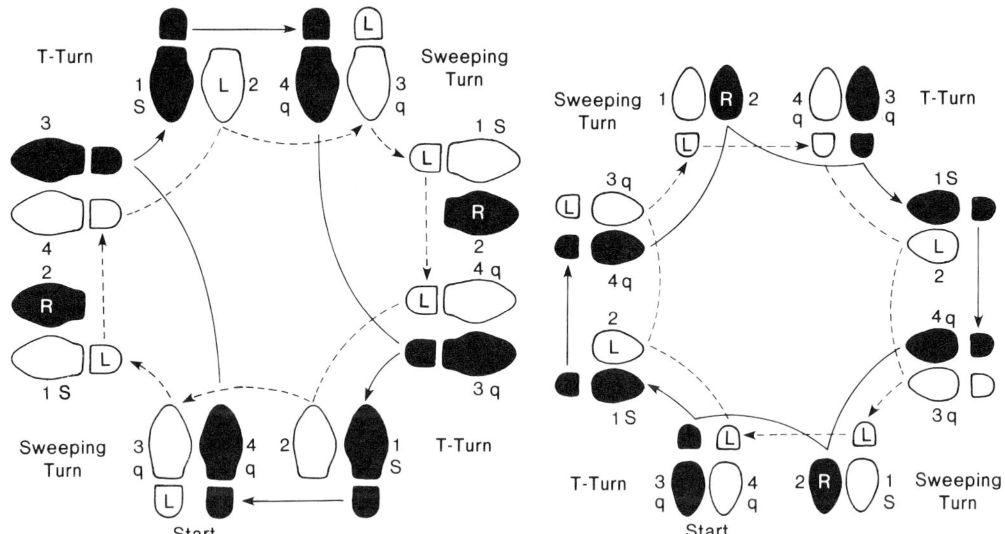

Figure 2.8. Left box turn

Step	Foot	Directional Cue	Count	Timing Cue	Comments
Forward Box Turn (¼)—interrelate with steps 2, 3 and 4 in woman's Magic Left Turn					
1	L	Fwd	1–2	S	Arc-shaped 4th pos. fwd step with toe leading ¼ CCW turn ct 2-tch R ft bsd L. "Sweeping Turn."
2	R	Sd	3	q	Directly to R sd
3	L	Tog	4	q	
Backward Box Turn (¼)—interrelate with Steps 2, 3 and 4 in man's Magic Left Turn					
1	R	Bwd	1–2	S	Turn R ft ¼ CCW first then body follows Ct 2-tch L ft bsd R. "T-Turn."
2	L	Sd	3	q	Directly to R sd
3	R	Tog	4	q	

Note: Man completes the full box turn by repeating one forward and one backward box turn. The woman's part is the natural opposite; as in the box step basic, the woman begins with the backward step pattern.

Pivot Turns (Magic Rhythm)

This continuous turning motion should be planned to the equivalent of magic timing or a series of six counts; i.e., the first two slow steps require four counts, and the next two quick steps will be equal to one magic step. The remainder of the quicks should be in groups of six. Too many turns will result in dizziness—focus on a certain spot as the turns are executed to alleviate the condition. There is a tendency for novices to limit their movement to a small CW circle, but eventually they should attempt to travel in direction of dance with their pivots.

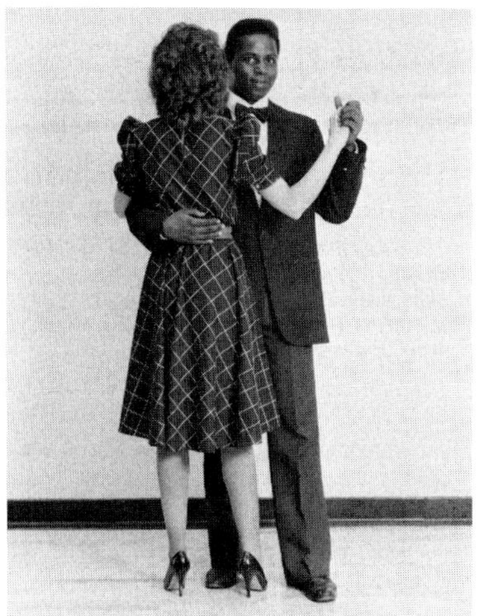

Figure 2.9. Pivot turn

Step	Foot	Directional Cue	Count	Timing Cue	Comments
Man's Part					
1	L	Fwd	1–2	S	Either basic closed or conversation position
2	R	Fwd	3–4	S	
3	L	L Frt	5	q	$\frac{1}{2}$ to $\frac{3}{4}$ turn on ball of ft, CW across dir. of dance
4	R	Fwd	6	q	R ft always step fwd in between partner's feet
5–10	L, R	Out, Fwd	7–12	qs	Continue turns as in steps 3 and 4 (ft in 2nd pos.)

Step	Foot	Directional Cue	Count	Timing Cue	Comments

Note: The woman's part is the natural opposite with the exception of step three, in which she also steps fwd so that her R ft is close to the man's R ft. This produces a "dovetailed" effect by each dancer stepping in between the partner's feet. This position is maintained throughout the pivots, and also all four feet should be kept in a straight line. Since the man always steps outward with his L, the woman always steps fwd with her R ft. Since the man always steps fwd with his R ft, the woman always steps outward with her L ft. Keep the hips close, but lean slightly bwd above the waist.

Woman's Part

Step	Foot	Directional Cue	Count	Timing Cue	Comments
1	R	Bwd	1–2	S	Either basic closed pos. or conversation pos.
2	L	Bwd	3–4	S	
3	R	Fwd	5	q	R ft always steps fwd between partner's ft
4	L	L Frt	6	q	½ turn on ball of ft, CW across dir. of dance
5–10	R,L	Fwd, Out	7–12	qs	Continue turns as in steps 3 and 4 with ft in 2nd pos.

Suggested Sequence: (man faces direction of dance to start)

2 box steps (complete)

1 left box turn (complete)

4 forward magic steps

4 backward magic steps

¾ magic left turn (the man faces out, the woman faces in to center)

3 swing steps (progressing in line of dance)

3 dip or corté steps

3 conversation steps (progressing in line of dance)

1 pivot turn series (starting with two slows in conversation position and manuevering on the pivots to face line of dance)

Suggested Musical Selections:

"New York, New York," vocalist—Frank Sinatra, Reprise Records, Warner Bros. Records Inc.

"Stardust" by Memo Bernabei and his Band, Windsor 4-541 B, Ballroom Dance Series.

"Stayin' Alive" RS 885 and/or "Night Fever" RS 889, by the BeeGees—Original Movie Soundtrack of Saturday Night Fever, RSO Records, Inc.

waltz

3

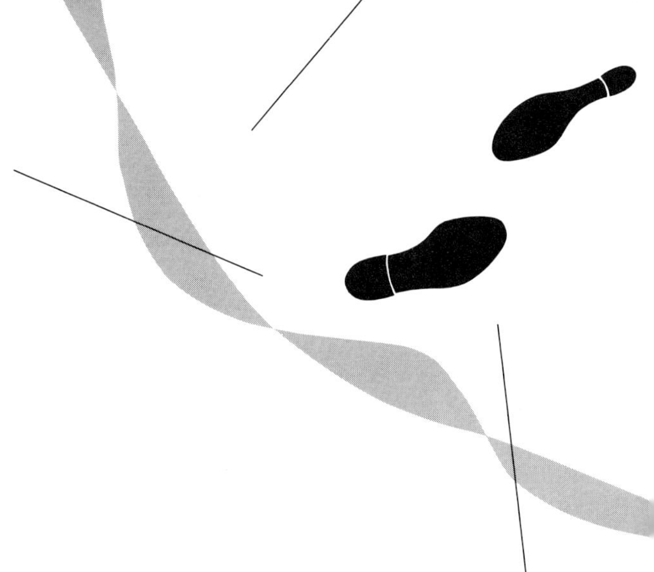

The waltz, the oldest of the ballroom dances, is credited with the introduction of the basic closed-couple dance position. France and Italy claim that the waltz originated in the Volta, which was a round dance of the late 1500s. It incorporated simple hand-holding in a circle and rough and rowdy triple-time turning movements. Two centuries later, Germany's and Austria's peasant dances, named after Joseph Ländlers, emphasized the term waltzers, which meant gliding and/or sliding. The new waltz position was met with great opposition at first and caused furor in the English ballrooms. The acceptance and eventual immortality of the waltz was due to Johann Strauss, an Austrian who composed very fast waltz music known as Viennese waltzes. Later, the slow waltz was adopted by the Americans and became known as the American style.

Timing

The waltz is the only ballroom dance that has $\frac{3}{4}$ rhythm. The basic step pattern consists of three steps which receive one count each. The basic timing should be cued as "1–2–3" or "quick, quick, quick." The leading foot will alternate and should be accented with body weight at the beginning of each measure. The waltz tempo can be fast, medium or slow, but the medium version is suggested when considering music for the beginner.

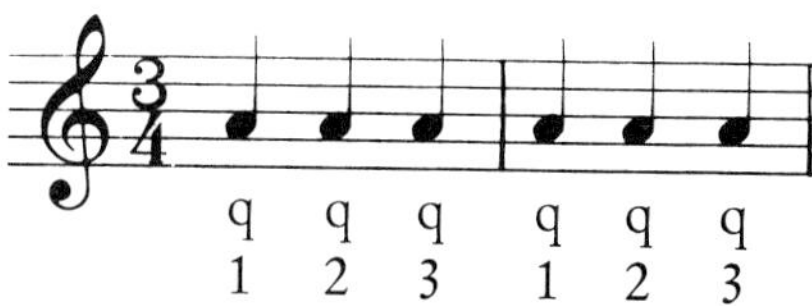

Figure 3.1. Waltz rhythmic pattern

Styling

The light and airy quality for which the waltz is renowned is related to its specific style. The waltz exaggerates a "rise and fall" effect that is present throughout the basic step pattern. On count one, the leading foot is flat on the floor, and the knee is bent (the cue word is "down" or "flat"). On counts two and three, the change is made to a high level so that foot is raised to the ball. The heels do not touch the floor (the cue words are "up, up"), and the knees are straight but not stiff. This results in an illusion of weightlessness and should be introduced after the novice feels confident about the basic step pattern.

Basic Step

The basic step of the waltz is the box step. It is the same as the basic box step of the fox-trot with these exceptions: (1) there are no slow (two-count) steps; therefore, a touch of the unweighted foot will not be incorporated, and (2) the rise and fall styling of the waltz is different from fox-trot styling. The woman's part is in natural opposition to the man's part. The fox-trot and waltz are closely interrelated as smooth dances.

The Box Step

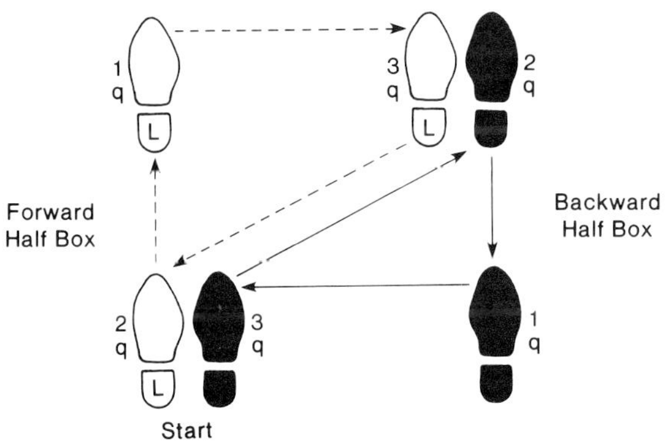

Figure 3.2. Box step, man

Step	Foot	Directional Cue	Count	Timing Cue	Comments
Forward Half Box					
1	L	Fwd	1	q	"down" or "flat"
2	R	Sd	2	q	"up," R ft follows a diagonal line to R sd
3	L	Tog	3	q	"up"

Step	Foot	Directional Cue	Count	Timing Cue	Comments
Backward Half Box					
1	R	Bwd	1	q	"down" or "flat"
2	L	Sd	2	q	"up," L ft follows a diagonal line to L sd
3	R	Tog	3	q	"up"

Note: As in the fox-trot basic box step, the man starts with the forward half box, and the woman starts with the backward half box. Then they alternate.

Variations (in order of difficulty)

Hesitation

Step	Foot	Directional Cue	Count	Timing Cue	Comments
Forward					
1	L	Fwd	1	q	"down," sl bent knee
2	R	Tch	2	q	"up," no wt chg, straighten knee (var—swing leg fwd)
3	(L)	Ho	3	q	Hold
Backward					
1	R	Bwd	1	q	"down", sl bent knee
2	L	Tch	2	q	"up," no wt chg, straighten knee (var—swing leg bwd)
3	R	Ho	3	q	Hold

Note: There is little movement in the hesitation. It is a simple method of keeping time. It can also be performed to either or both sides.

Balance

Step	Foot	Directional Cue	Count	Timing Cue	Comments
Forward					
1	L	Fwd	1	q	"down"
2	R	Fwd	2	q	"up" on both ft, R ft wt chg
3	L	IP	3	q	"down" to heels of both ft

Step	Foot	Directional Cue	Count	Timing Cue	Comments
Backward					
1	R	Bwd	1	q	"down"
2	L	Bwd	2	q	"up" on both ft, L ft wt chg
3	R	IP	3	q	"down" to heels of both ft

Note: This is similar to the hesitation except on steps two and three the weight is changed alternately. This variation of the basic box step can also be performed to either or both sides.

Progressive Step (Man's part)

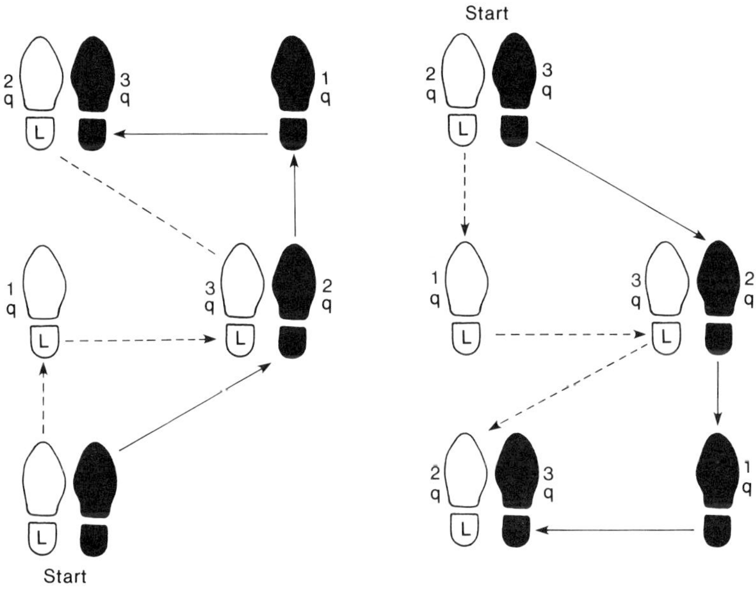

a. Forward progressive (Man)

b. Backward progressive (Man)

Figure 3.3. Progressive step, man

Step	Foot	Directional Cue	Count	Timing Cue	Comments
Forward (2 successive Half Boxes)					
1	L	Fwd	1	q	"down"
2	R	Sd	2	q	"up," R ft follows a diagonal line to R sd
3	L	Tog	3	q	"up"

Step	Foot	Directional Cue	Count	Timing Cue	Comments
4	R	Fwd	1	q	"down"
5	L	Sd	2	q	"up," L ft follows a diagonal line to L sd
6	R	Tog	3	q	"up"
Backward (2 successive Half Boxes)					
1	L	Bwd	1	q	"down"
2	R	Sd	2	q	"up," R ft follows a diagonal line to R sd
3	L	Tog	3	q	"up"
4	R	Bwd	1	q	"down"
5	L	Sd	2	q	"up," L ft follows a diagonal line to L sd
6	R	Tog	3	q	"up"

Note: The progressive step can be performed in a series of several forward and several backward box steps.

Variation: A type of advanced follow-through technique can be attempted on this step pattern by omitting the "side-togethers" and simply walking forward ("down," "up," "up") on all steps (man's part). This is sometimes called the pursuit step.

Progressive Step (Woman's part)

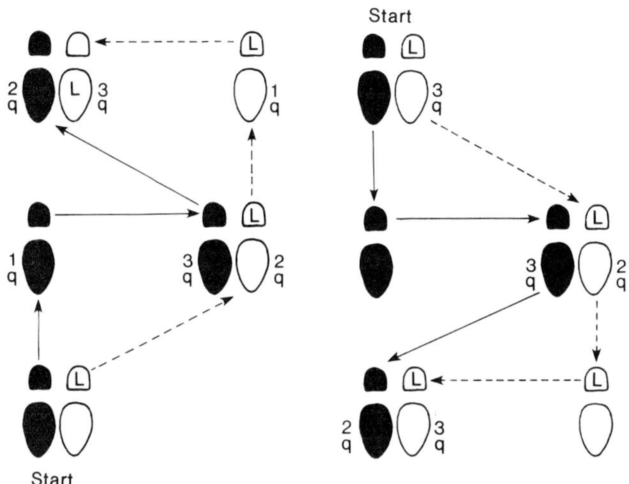

a. Forward progressive (Woman)   b. Backward progressive (Woman)

Figure 3.4. Progressive step, woman

Step	Foot	Directional Cue	Count	Timing Cue	Comments
Forward (2 successive Half Boxes)					
1	R	Bwd	1	q	"down"
2	L	Sd	2	q	"up," L ft follows a diagonal line to L sd
3	R	Tog	3	q	"up"
4	L	Bwd	1	q	"down"
5	R	Sd	2	q	"up," R ft follows a diagonal line to R sd
6	L	Tog	3	q	"up"
Backward (2 successive Half Boxes)					
1	R	Fwd	1	q	"down"
2	L	Sd	2	q	"up," L ft follows a diagonal line to L sd
3	R	Tog	3	q	"up"
4	L	Fwd	1	q	"down"
5	R	Sd	2	q	"up," R ft follows a diagonal line to R sd
6	L	Tog	3	q	"up"

Turns

Left Box Turn

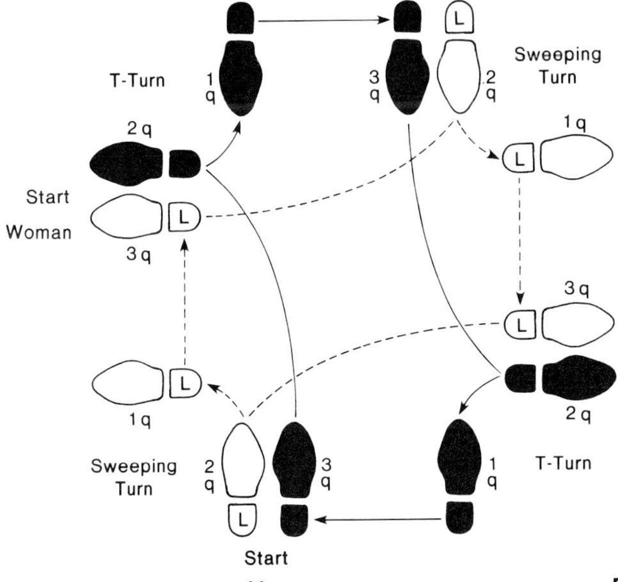

Figure 3.5. Left box turn

Step	Foot	Directional Cue	Count	Timing Cue	Comments
Forward Box Turn (¼)					
1	L	Fwd	1	q	Arc-shaped 4th pos. fwd step with toe leading ¼ CCW. "Sweeping turn", "down"
2	R	Sd	2	q	R ft follows a diagonal line to rt sd. "up"
3	L	Tog	3	q	"up"
Backward Box Turn (¼)					
1	R	Bwd	1	q	Turn R ft ¼ CCW first. "T-Turn", "down"
2	L	Sd	2	q	L ft follows a diagonal line to lt sd. "up"
3	R	Tog	3	q	"up"

Note: Man completes the full box turn by repeating one forward and one backward box turn. As in the box step basic, the woman begins with the backward step pattern. The waltz left box turn is similar to the fox-trot left box turn, but the timing is different.

Variation: The left box turn can be modified to develop interesting step patterns.

> *Hesitation and Left Box Turn Combination:* This variation consists of one hesitation step pattern (no turn is required), which is followed by one backward left box turn (man's part). It is the waltz equivalent of the magic left turn in fox-trot. Repeat three times to face original direction.

> *Cross Variation:* As in the fox-trot magic left turn, the waltz equivalent can incorporate a cross, performed in conversation position, on the last step of step pattern. (Hence, this variation can also be used on the last step of the backward left box turn—man's part—and can serve as a nice transition to the next step pattern.)

Underarm Turn

The man's part for the underarm turn requires the waltz box-step footwork. His lead indications are very important for this step pattern. He lifts his left arm and her right arm (respective hands joined loosely) up to arch position, and he uses his right hand (near her left shoulder blade) to lightly push her under the arch. As he performs the forward half box, she walks under the arch in a small CW circle, R (q, "down"), L (q, "up"), R (q, "up") and returns to face him directly to complete the box step with a forward half box.

Suggested Sequence: (similar to suggested sequence in fox-trot for simplicity)

2 box steps (complete)

1 left box turn (complete)

4 forward progressive steps

4 backward progressive steps

1 hesitation and left box turn combination (complete)—magic left turn equivalent

4 balances and/or hesitations (in place)

Suggested Musical Selections:

"Melody of Love" by Al Martino, Starline—a subsidiary of Capitol Records, 6108.

"Moon River" by Memo Bernabei and his Band, Windsor 4-541A, Ballroom Dance Series.

"Shadow Waltz," Hoctor, #617.

"Alice Blue Gown," Hoctor.

tango
4

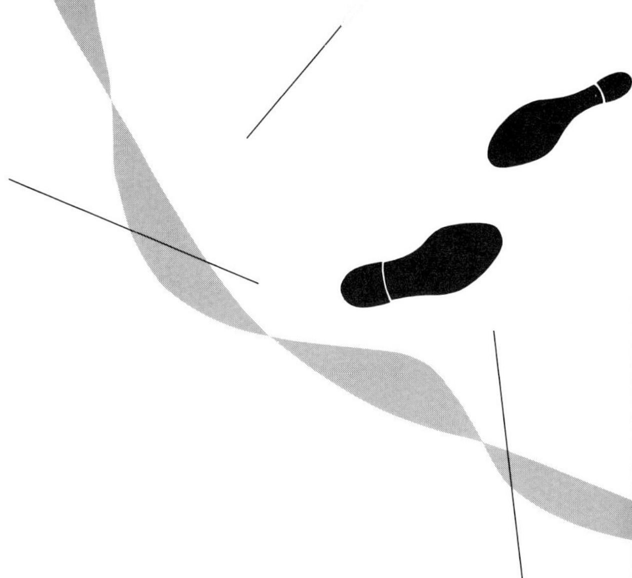

The origin of the tango is diversified. Some authorities claim that the tango was created in Spain, where solo dancers performed a gypsy Iberian dance that resembled the heel-beating, sharp staccato, $\frac{2}{4}$ rhythm of the flamenco dance.

Around the beginning of the twentieth century, the lower classes of Buenos Aires developed a dance in which the participants wore gaucho clothing. This Argentine tango was soon introduced in Paris and then London, where the afternoon "tango teas" became fashionable. At first the Americans adopted the French version, but Vernon and Irene Castle promoted the Argentine tango and stabilized the many influences on the American style. Rudolph Valentino also helped to popularize the tango in America. It became known as a romantic, sophisticated dance.

Timing

Tango music is composed of obvious phrases of eight measures each. One tango basic step in $\frac{4}{4}$ time will require a subphrase of two measures or eight counts.

It is cued as "slow, slow, quick, quick, slow" or "1–2, 3–4, 5–6, 7–8 Tan-go close." As familiarity with the tango increases, the novice will learn to recognize the unmistakable rhythm and sound of the tango music.

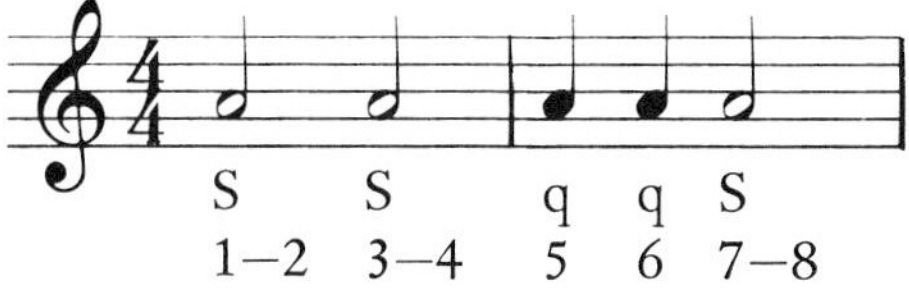

Figure 4.1. Tango rhythmic pattern

Styling

Tango is a well-controlled Latin dance in which the two dancers move together as one. Emphasis is placed upon leg motions that drive forward or backward from the hips to produce long, low (bent knees), flat-footed steps. The "tan-go close" portion of the basic step ends with an abrupt halt which is characteristic in the styling of the dance. In Argentina, the tango's original name was "baile con cortë," which meant the "dance with a stop."

Another styling technique that is identified with the tango is a slow, low pivot step (usually a half-pivot), which could be performed as either a "hook" or as a "fan." They are both concerned with the action of the free leg during the pivot.

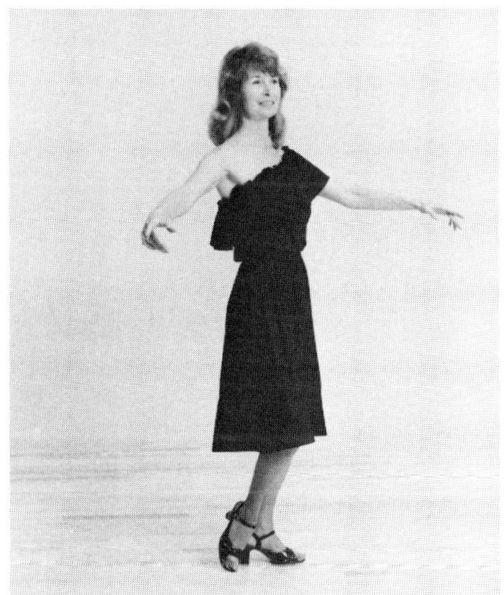

Figure 4.2. Hook position

In a "hook," the ankle of the free leg is pressed behind and slightly above the ankle of the supporting leg to form a 90-degree angle (or a modified third foot position with the weight-free ankle elevated and knee flexed).

In a "fan," the free leg is straight and directed diagonally outward with toes pointed. The knee of the supporting leg is flexed to lower the dancer's center of gravity. Since the fan step patterns are more complex, they will be treated separately at the end of the tango variations.

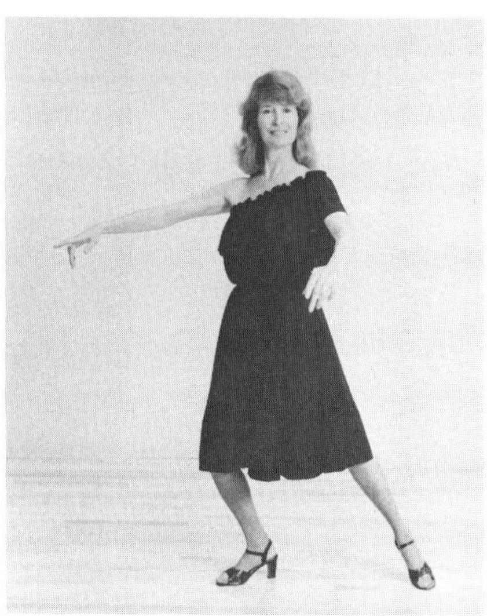

Figure 4.3. Fan position

Basic Step

The Tango is known as the Latin fox-trot, and their basic steps are similar. An interrelationship also occurs between the forward half box step in waltz and the "tan-go close;" i.e., they both involve Fwd, Sd, Tog.

Step	Foot	Directional Cue	Count	Timing Cue	Comments
Man's Part					
1	L	Fwd	1–2	S	Close body contact from the shoulders to the knees
2	R	Fwd	2–4	S	
3	L	Fwd	5	q	The L ft initiates the break or tan-go close
4	R	Sd	6	q	R ft follows a diag. line to R sd Man's lead—draw R hand & elbow to R
5	L	Tog	7–8	S	L ft should draw slowly (for a full ct) to the R ft and hold ct 8

Note: Since there is no weight change on the draw (last step), the man starts the next step pattern with his left foot. The woman's part is in natural opposition.

Step	Foot	Directional Cue	Count	Timing Cue	Comments
Lady's Part					
1	R	Bwd	1–2	S	Close body contact from the shoulders to the knees
2	L	Bwd	3–4	S	
3	R	Bwd	5	q	The R ft initiates the break

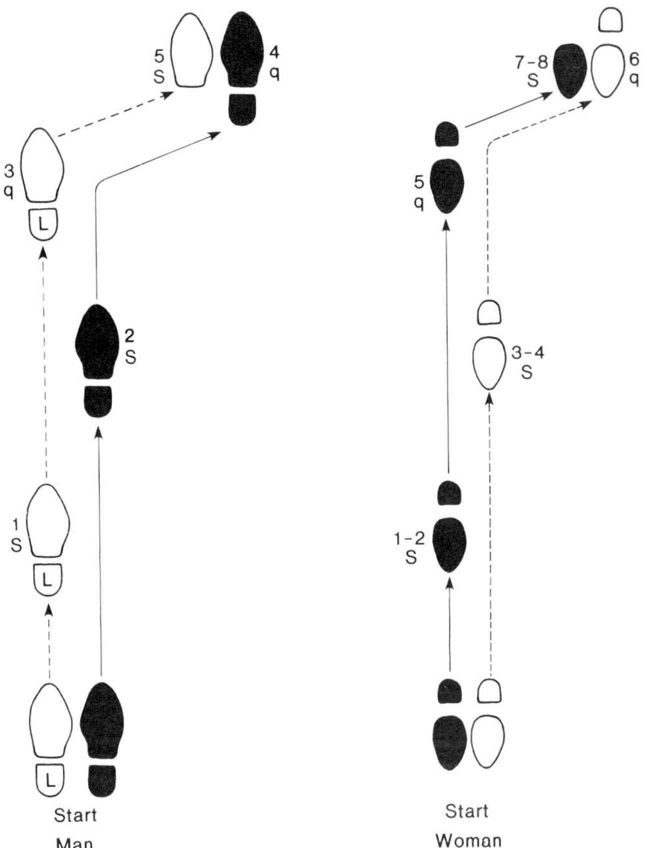

Figure 4.4. Tango basic step

Step	Foot	Directional Cue	Count	Timing Cue	Comments
4	L	Sd	6	q	L ft follows a diag. line to L sd
5	R	Tog	7–8	S	R ft draws slowly for a full ct to the L ft and hold for ct 8

Backward Basic Step: The directional cues for steps 1, 2 and 3 are reversed to be backward steps for the man and forward steps for the woman.

Note: The last portion of each basic step pattern, the tango close, will move the couple toward the outside wall. In order to counter this effect, it is necessary to learn variations that will change the direction of travel, such as the right parallel basic step, turns and the conversation step.

Parallel (Rt): Assume Rt parallel position on steps 1 and 2 and a short step on step 3 to return immediately to closed-couple dance position.

Turns

Quarter Turn (on the tango close)
The quarter turn is similar to the left box turn in waltz.

Step	Foot	Directional Cue	Count	Timing Cue	Comments
Man's Part					
1	L	Fwd	1–2	S	
2	R	Fwd	3–4	S	
3	L	Fwd	5	q	Arc-shaped 4th pos. fwd step with toe leading ¼ CCW turn
4	R	Sd	6	q	R ft follows a diagonal line to R sd.
5	L	Dr	7–8	S	Draw L ft to R ft (no wt chg)
Woman's Part					
1	R	Bwd	1–2	S	
2	L	Bwd	3–4	S	
3	R	Bwd	5	q	Turn R ft ¼ CCW first, then body follows.
4	L	Sd	6	q	L ft follows a diagonal line to R sd.
5	R	Dr	7–8	S	Draw R ft to L ft (no wt chg)

Quarter Turn with Cross Step

Step	Foot	Directional Cue	Count	Timing Cue	Comments
Man's Part					
1	L	Sd	1–2	S	
2	R	Fwd	3–4	S	Assume conversation pos. and step through with R ft
3	L	Fwd	5	q	Arc-shaped 4th pos. fwd step with toe leading ¼ CCW turn (Lead—fwd motion of fingers of R hand)
4	R	Sd	6	q	
5	L	Dr	7–8	S	Draw R ft to L ft (no wt chg)
Woman's Part					
1	R	Sd	1–2	S	
2	L	Fwd	3–4	S	Conversation pos., step through with L ft and ½ CCW (hook) on ball of L ft to face partner
3	R	Mnvr	5	q	
4	L	Sd	6	q	
5	R	Dr	7–8	S	Draw R ft to the L ft

Variations

Conversation Step

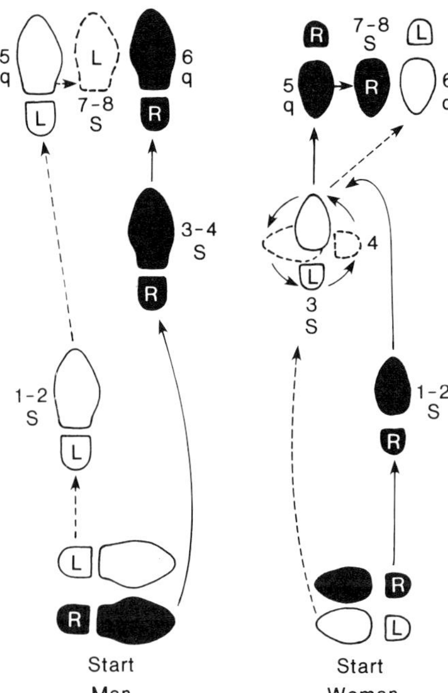

Figure 4.5. Conversation step

Step	Foot	Directional Cue	Count	Timing Cue	Comments
Man's Part					
1	L	Fwd	1–2	S	On ct 1, assume conversation pos. (sharp lead with heel of R hand, L arm straightens and head turns).
2	R	Fwd	3–4	S	R ft follows through (finish step with sharp Fwd movement of R hand so the woman will face toward him)
3	L	Fwd	5	q	Short step in same direction (Closed-couple dance position, but facing ¼ Lt turn from orig. dir.)
4	R	Sd	6	q	
5	L	Dr	7–8	S	Draw L ft to the R (no wt chg)

Step	Foot	Directional Cue	Count	Timing Cue	Comments
Woman's Part					
1	R	Fwd	1–2	S	On ct 1, sharply assume conversation pos. (R arm straightens and head turns).
2	L	Fwd	3–4	S	L ft follows through (after stepping, man's lead will turn her on ball of her L ft to hook and face him sharply).
3	R	Bwd	5	q	Short step (closed-couple dance position)
4	L	Sd	6	q	
5	R	Dr	7–8	S	Draw R ft to the L ft (no wt chg)

Note: The conversation step is an integral part of the tango and a favorite step pattern of ballroom dancers. A simplified version is to face partner on ct 5 to finish the tango-close in starting position.

Medio Corte or Dip (Man's Part)

Step	Foot	Directional Cue	Count	Timing Cue	Comments
1	L	Fwd	1	q	Short step
2	R	IP	2	q	Wt chg slightly bwd to R ft
3	L	Bwd	3–4	S	Long step, dip with L leg bent, R leg str., torso erect
4	R	IP	5–6	S	Recover by changing wt to R ft
(Repeat)					
5	L	Fwd	7	q	Short step
6	R	IP	8	q	Wt chg slightly bwd to R ft (rocking action)
7	L	Bwd	9–10	S	Long step, dip, R ft maintains contact with the floor
8	R	IP	11–12	S	Recover rocking fwd to R ft
(Ending: Tan-go close)					
9	L	Fwd	13	q	
10	R	Sd	14	q	
11	L	Dr	15–16	S	

Note: Variations such as the medio corté must be planned in multiples of eight counts, otherwise the step pattern will not concur with the musical subphrase. (The basic tango step also has eight counts.) The woman's part is in direct opposition to that of the man's. On the third and seventh steps or dips, her R leg knee is flexed and over the instep and her L leg is straight as she lunges forward. (The fox-trot corté was a similar version of the dip.)

Fan Steps

La Puerta (Parallel Fan)

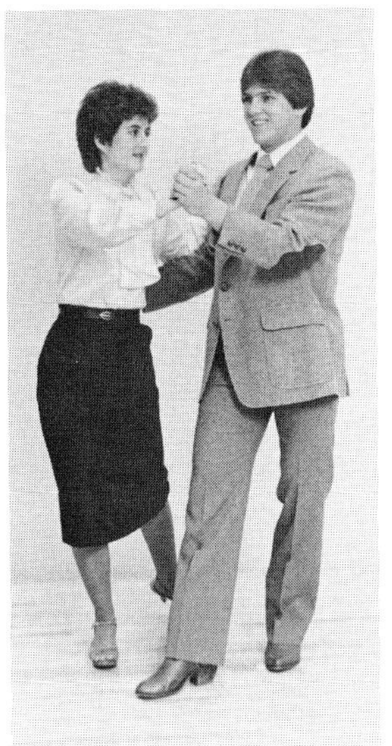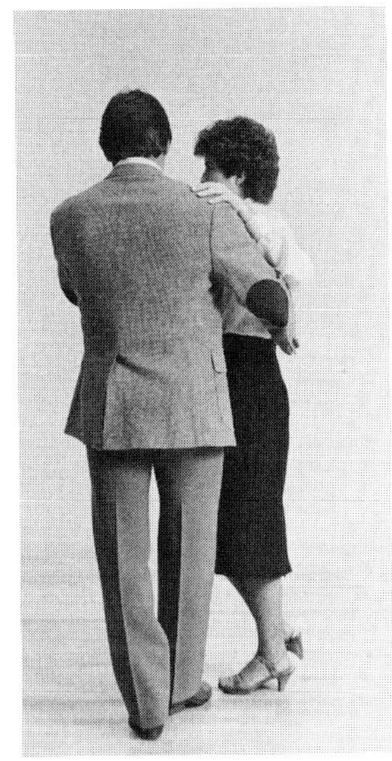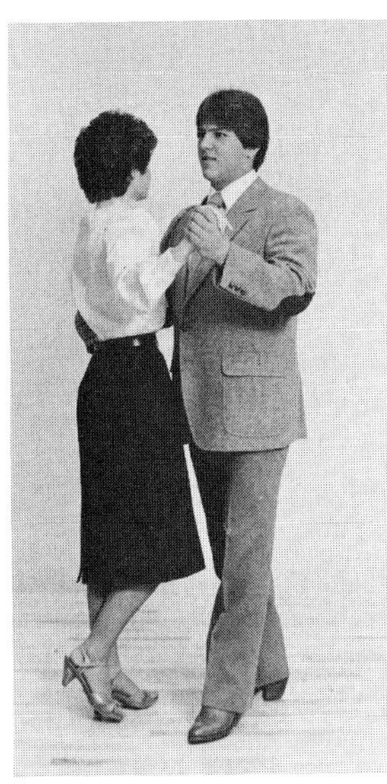

Figure 4.6. La Puerta

La Puerta means "the door" in Spanish. The man's part has the same foot pattern as the medio corté, but the lead indications are different. The woman performs the "fans."

Step	Foot	Directional Cue	Count	Timing Cue	Comments
Man's Part					
1	L	Fwd	1	q	Short step
2	R	IP	2	q	Wt chg (slightly bwd) to R ft
3	L	Bwd	3–4	S	Long step with slight dip. Also step slightly to the left. Lead-R (bent) elbow and hand forcefully to the right side and bwd through parallel pos.
4	R	IP	5–6	S	Recover (wt chg) to R ft. Lead-R hand describes ½ CW circle to face open pos., palm fwd, and follow through extending arm. Then flex wrist twd him forcefully (to turn woman twd him; she remains to his R)

Step	Foot	Directional Cue	Count	Timing Cue	Comments
5–8 Repeat			7–12		
9	L	Fwd	13	q	Closed-couple dance pos. (¼ turn is appropriate).
10	R	Sd	14	q	
11	L	Dr	15–16	S	Draw L ft to R ft
Woman's Part					
1	R	Bwd	1	q	Short step
2	L	IP	2	q	Wt chg slightly fwd to the L
3	R	Fwd	3–4	S	Long step fwd in parallel pos.; at end of step, perform a fan (wt on R ft, ½ pivot with L leg str. out) to face open pos.
4	L	Fwd	5–6	S	Long step fwd; at end of step, perform a hook or fan (wt on L ft, ½ pivot) to face parallel pos.
5–8 Repeat			7–12		
9	R	Bwd	13	q	Closed-couple dance pos. (¼ turn is appropriate)
10	L	Sd	14	q	
11	R	Dr	15–16	S	Draw R ft to L ft

Butterfly Fan Step (Open Position Fan)

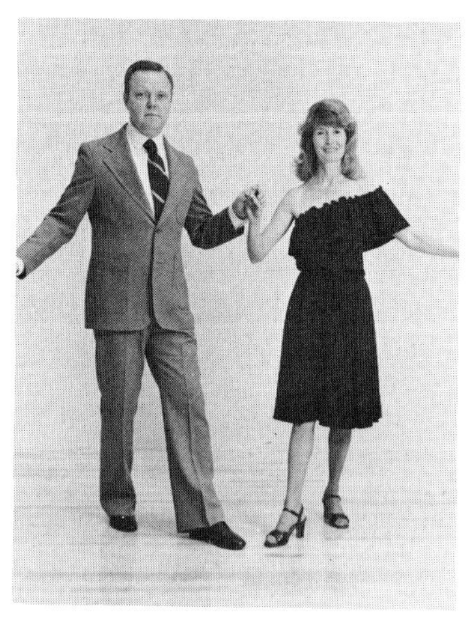
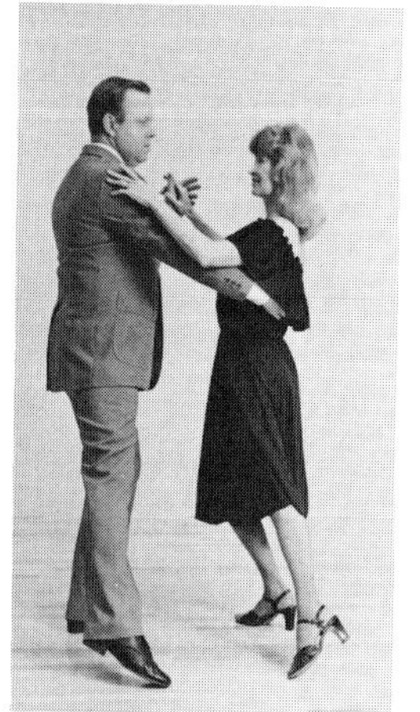
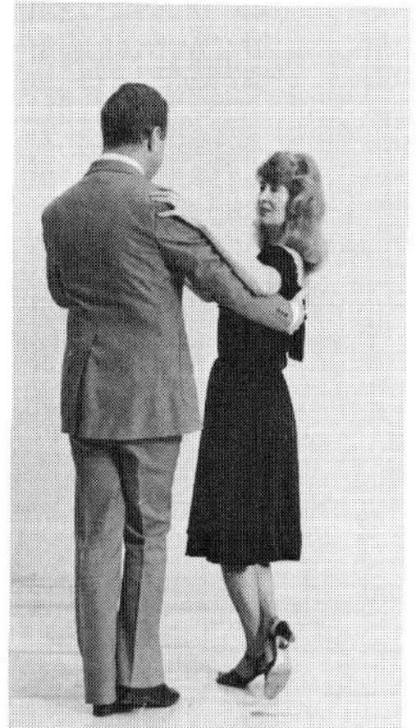

Figure 4.7. Butterfly fan

Step	Foot	Directional Cue	Count	Timing Cue	Comments
Man's Part					
1	L	Fwd	1–2	S	On ct 1, assume conversation pos.
2	R	Fwd	3–4	S	R ft follows through (turn ft slightly to R)
3	L	Fwd	5	q	Release R arm (from woman) to full open pos. and then perform a ½ CW turn, taking woman's R hand in man's L hand (facing opposite of conversation direction)
4	R	Sd	6	q	Ft in 2nd pos.
5	L	Dr	7–8	S	Draw L ft to R ft in full open pos. (no wt chg)
6	L	Fwd	9–10	S	(Opposite of original conversation dir.) Take wt on L ft and perform a ½ CCW Fan pivot twd partner
7	R	Fwd	11–12	S	(Original conversation dir. to complete a conversation step as previously described
8	L	Fwd	13	q	returning to basic closed couple dance pos.—with ¼ CCW turn if
9	R	Sd	14	q	possible.)
10	L	Dr	15–16	S	Draw L ft to R ft in closed pos.
Woman's Part					
1	R	Fwd	1–2	S	On ct 1, assume conversation pos.
2	L	Fwd	3–4	S	L ft follows thru
3	R	Fwd	5	q	Release L arm from man to full open pos. and then perform a ½ CCW turn, taking man's L hand in woman's R hand.
4	L	Sd	6	q	Ft in 2nd pos.
5	R	Dr	7–8	S	Draw R ft to L ft in full open pos. with no wt chg
6	R	Fwd	9–10	S	Take wt on R ft and perform a ½ CW Fan pivot twd partner
7	L	Fwd	11–12	S	Take wt on L ft and perform a ½ CCW Hook pivot twd partner
8	R	Bwd	13	q	Complete a tan-go close
9	L	Sd	14	q	
10	R	Dr	15–16	S	

Suggested Sequence:

4 forward basic steps
4 backward basic steps
4 conversation steps (first and third toward center of circle)
2 medio corté
2 la puerta
1 butterfly fan step

Suggested Musical Selections:

"Derecho Viejo," Valdesari-Arolas, Hoctor H-678B, Tango.
"Inspiration," N. E. Paulos, Hoctor H-678A, Tango.
"Kiss of Fire," Hoctor, #689.
"Tango of Hearts," Hoctor, #689.
"Orchids in the Moonlight," Hoctor, #1631.
"Poema," Hoctor, #1631.
"La Comparsita," Hoctor, #1644A.

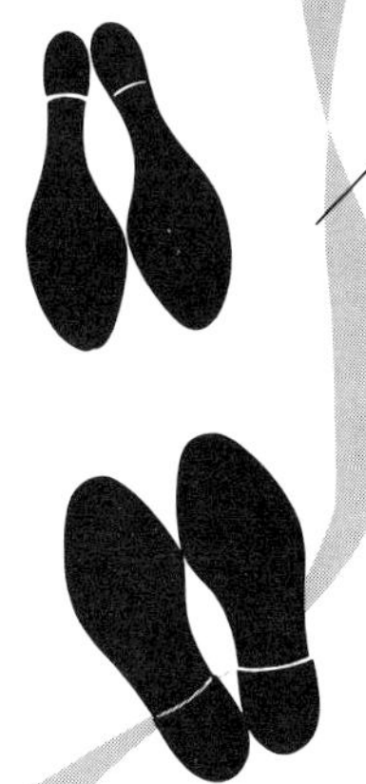

part
3

rhythm dances

The remainder of the ballroom dances that cannot be classified as smooth dances are known as rhythm dances. This category includes the swing, polka and similar regional dances, samba, merengue, mambo, cha-cha and rumba. These dances, with the exception of the swing and polka, are of Latin origin. Each dance has inherent styling techniques that differentiate it from the other dances. However, all of the rhythm dances have common characteristics that identify them as part of this classification: the man's lead indications originate in his upper torso and are transmitted through his arms and hands, and the steps are small (about the size of your foot), flat and close to the floor.

The rhythm dances add scope and dimension to the dancer's repertoire. Dancers will derive hours of enjoyment and satisfaction from participating in these versatile and fascinating rhythm dances.

swing
5

In the early decades of the 1900s, the conventional musically-scored sounds of ragtime induced the extemporaneous jazz style, which evolved into a new combination of both melody and short outbursts of improvisation to become known as swing. Benny Goodman, the "King of Swing," developed the syncopated swing rhythm, which accents the off-beat counts of two and four in $\frac{4}{4}$ time. The Fox-trot was not adaptable to this new trend in timing, and the beat was too invigorating to ignore, so the development of new dances was justified.

The lindy hop, named in honor of pilot Charles Lindberg in 1927, was the first of the swing-type dances. A decade later, in Harlem, a new form was generated, called the jitterbug (named because the participants looked like "jittery bugs"). It introduced two major changes: (1) the breakaway or solo part, which originated in African dances and (2) the "air steps" or acrobatics. The shag was a version that involved kicks and stomps. Each subsequent decade had its popular swing-style dance: the boogie-woogie (a Negro term), rock 'n roll, solo fad dances, disco, country-swing, and rock. These dance crazes were accepted by the young and agile, but not necessarily by the sophisticates, who preferred to remain demure. They developed a subdued, durable, ballroom-style rendition that became known as swing.

Timing

Swing rhythm was derived from the fox-trot magic step. A six-count basic step is common to both. The single-time version (slow, slow quick, quick) is the easiest but can be adapted to the faster swing music. Double-time (six quicks) doubles the emphasis of syncopation by stepping stronger on counts two and four. Triple-time (quick 'n quick, quick 'n quick, quick, quick) involves triplets, or three steps taken in the count of two, and therefore requires a slower swing music. Most variations will stress the use of the triple-time rhythm.

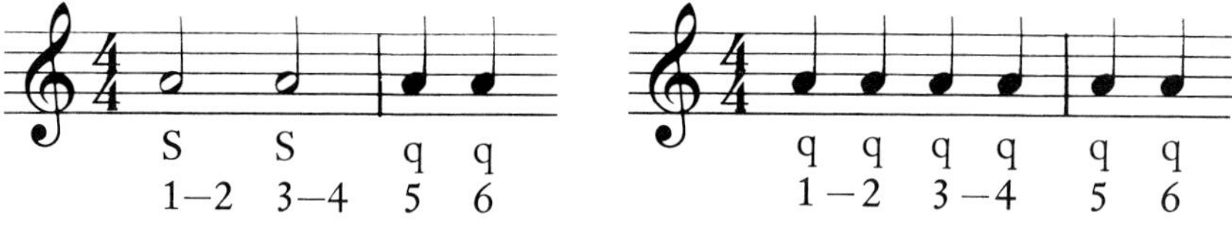

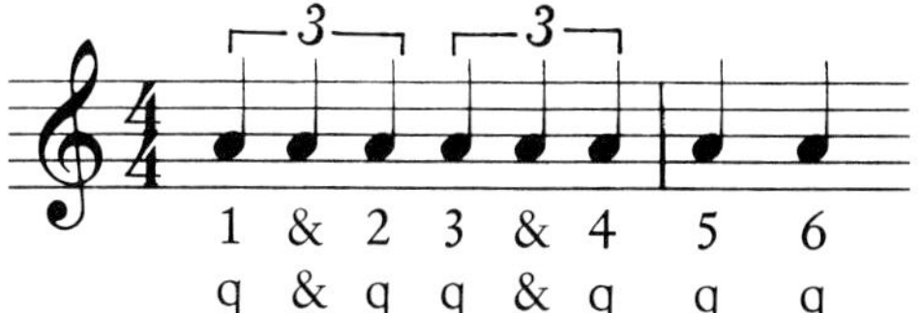

Figure 5.1.

Styling

Swing has a free-style quality of exuberant, quick movements. Its rotational patterns require a semiopen dance position and a modified hand hold, which is used only in swing-style dancing.

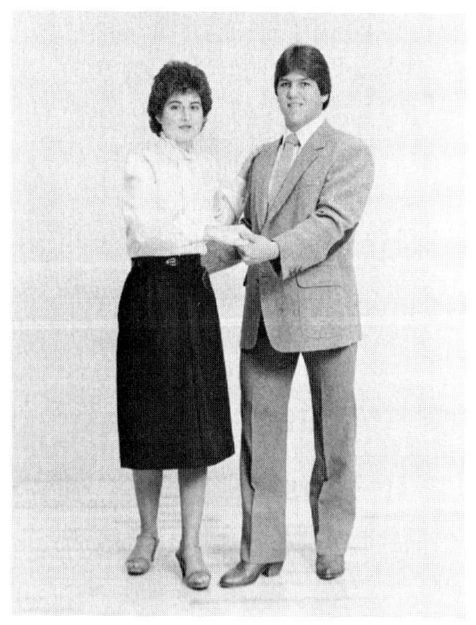

Figure 5.2. Swing position

Directions for the swing hand hold: (Semiopen position)

1. The man's left hand is extended with the palm up and the thumb lifted upward.
2. The man rotates his hand inward to point his fingers toward his partner.

3. The woman places her hand with the palm down over the palmside of his fingers and also points her fingers toward him.
4. The man firmly places his thumb diagonally across the back of her hand and her fingers.

The joined hands and their respective forearms should maintain a firm resistance so that positions can be changed responsively. The elbow remains firmly flexed, even on the break step (counts five and six), in which the couple maintains the front hand hold but turns outward to a side-to-side position. The break step is the only constant in the three types of basic six-count steps. Throughout most of the variations, the knees should be flexed to absorb the shock and allow easy, informal motions. It requires balance and coordination through fast changes of weight in the footwork.

Basic Steps (Man's Part)

Step	Foot	Directional Cue	Count	Timing Cue	Comments
Single-time					
1	L	Sd	1–2	S	The off-beat can be emphasized by brushing the free ft against the supporting ft on ct 2 (cue—"step, hit").
2	R	Sd	3–4	S	Same as above on ct 4.
3	L	Bwd	5	q	Rock away from partner by stepping with body wt firmly on the ball of the L ft, a few inches behind R ft. Do not drop to heel. (Cue—"break" or "rock")
4	R	IP	6	q	Shift wt evenly to fwd ft (cue—"step").
Double-time					
1	L	Tch	1	q	"Dig" or "touch" L ft (no wt) close to R, knees tog. Lead—dip L shoulder sl.
2	L	Sd	2	q	Now put wt on L ft, stepping out to sd about one-foot length. Emphasize ct 2.
3	R	Tch	3	q	"Dig" with R ft
4	R	Sd	4	q	Put wt on R ft, stepping out to R sd., accent ct 4.
5	L	Bwd	5	q	"Break." Turn outward, away from each other
6	R	IP	6	q	"Step." Turn toward each other

Step	Foot	Directional Cue	Count	Timing Cue	Comments
Triple-time					
First Half-Basic					
1	L	Sd	1	q	A triplet is three notes in the time of two. A triple-time step is three steps in the ct of two. "Flat"
2	R	Tog	&	'n	Still moving to the L sd, step on ball of R ft (chg of wt) "Ball"
3	L	Sd	2	q	Continue moving to L sd. "Flat"
Second Half-Basic					
4	R	Sd	3	q	Starting the second triple-time step, chg dir. to the R. "Flat"
5	L	Tog	&	'n	Take small steps throughout. "Ball"
6	R	Sd	4	q	"Flat"
Break Step					
7	L	Bwd	5	q	"Break." Turn outward, away from each other
8	R	IP	6	q	"Step." Turn toward each other

Note: Woman's part is in natural opposition, except on the "break"—she steps bwd also.

Basic Steps (Woman's part)

Step	Foot	Directional Cue	Count	Timing Cue	Comments
Single-time					
1	R	Sd	1–2	S	Syncopate the rhythm by brushing the free ft against supporting ft on ct 2. Cue: "step, hit."
2	L	Sd	3–4	S	Repeat on ct 4.
3	R	Bwd	5	q	Rock away from partner by stepping with body wt firmly on the ball of R ft, a few inches behind L ft. Do not drop to heel. Cue: "break."
4	L	IP	6	q	Shift wt evenly to fwd ft. Cue: "step."
Double-time					
1	R	Tch	1	q	"Dig" or "touch" R ft (no wt) close to L, knees tog.

Step	Foot	Directional Cue	Count	Timing Cue	Comments
2	R	Sd	2	q	Place wt on R ft, stepping out to R sd about one-foot length. Stress ct 2.
3	L	Tch	3	q	"Dig" with L ft
4	L	Sd	4	q	Place wt on L ft, stepping out to L sd, accent on ct 4.
5	R	Bwd	5	q	"Break" or "rock." Turn outward, away from partner (conversation pos.).
6	L	IP	6	q	"Step." Turn toward partner.
Triple-time					
First Half-Basic					
1	R	Sd	1	q	This is the first of three steps in succession. Cue: "flat"
2	L	Tog	&	'n	Continue moving sl. to the R sd. Step on ball lf L ft with chg of wt. Cue: "Ball."
3	R	Sd	2	q	Last of the triple-time step to the R. Cue: "Flat."
Second Half-Basic					
4	L	Sd	3	q	Starting the second triple-time step, chg dir. to the L. Cue: "Flat."
5	R	Tog	&	'n	Take small steps throughout. Cue: "Ball."
6	L	Sd	4	q	Shift wt evenly. Cue: "Flat."
Break-Step					
7	R	Bwd	5	q	"Break" is the cue. Turn outward.
8	L	IP	6	q	"Step" is the cue. Turn toward partner.

Variations

Fundamentals

These are the basis for almost all variations in swing. Practice them diligently so that the movements will be fluid and natural.

Turning Basic

The dancers assume semiopen position to facilitate a clockwise turn to the right. (Swing and polka are the only dances that basically turn to the right.) The dancers turn (¼ to ½) together, facing each other in swing position, on the first half-basic of triple-time rhythm. (Single-time or double-time could also be used.) The man leads the step pattern by dropping his left shoulder slightly as he steps to the left, toward the woman, pivoting in a clockwise direction on the left foot. He continues his circular direction on the remainder of the two steps. The second half-basic is performed in place to face the partner directly. The break step completes the step pattern. Semiopen position is maintained throughout. The woman also moves in a clockwise direction, pivoting on the ball of the foot. Her part is in natural opposition to the man's part. (Cue words—"turn–2–3, in place–2–3, break step")

Throw-out (to Open Position)

The man's part is simply two basic steps (triple-time). He leads the throw-out by pushing the woman out to full open position with the heel of his right hand and extension of his left arm. The leads are given as the first step is taken, and the remainder of the basic step is completed in full open position. At the beginning of the second basic step, he leads the woman back to semiopen position by pulling his left arm (her right arm) downward toward him and resuming the remainder of the basic step. (Cue words—"out-or in–2–3, in place–2–3, break step")

The woman's part differs from the man's part. As he throws her out to full open position, she turns counter-clockwise about ½ (pivot on R ft) turn while performing her first half-basic. She should now be facing the same direction as the man. Her second half-basic and break step are done in place. On the first half-basic of the next step pattern, she resumes the original semiopen position by turning clockwise ½ (pivot on L ft) turn toward the man. She then completes the second half-basic and break step in place. (Cue words—"turn–2–3, in place–2–3, break step")

Underarm Turn

The man's part in the underarm turn is the same as that of the throw-out, except that the arch position is used on the first half-basic of each triple-time step. The man leads the underarm turn by pushing the woman with the heel of his right hand so that she will go under the arch formed by his left arm and her right arm. Her hand rotates inside of his hand on the turn. After completing the first basic step, the couple is in full open position. At the beginning of the second basic step, he makes an arch so that the woman can return in similar fashion to the original semiopen position. (Cue words—"arch–2–3, in place–2–3, break step")

The woman's part also differs from the throw-out only on the first half-basic of each basic step. As the man leads her into the first half-basic, she walks under the arch, turning slightly to her right or clockwise, to assume full open position and complete the first basic step in place. To return on the first half-basic of the second basic step, she turns counter-clockwise, under her own right arm, while moving to the right and backward as she turns to move toward the man. The second half-basic and break step are completed facing the original direction. (Cue words—"under–2–3, in place–2–3, break step")

Underarm Exchange

As part of the underarm turns, the underarm exchange adds the correct styling technique to the step pattern. The underarm exchange is incorporated only after the first basic step has been completed and the full open position has been attained. On the return underarm turn, the man and the woman simply add an exchange of places as they move across to each other's position. The man moves around the woman as she is turning under the arch. The underarm exchange can be performed any number of times in succession. The "get-out" is simply to move toward each other with a basic step to once again assume swing position or preferably to incorporate the turning basic step in the process.

Note: As the dancers exchange places, the man can also turn under his own left arm simultaneously with the woman.

Tuck Underarm Turn

The first half-basic of the underarm turn step pattern can be changed to add variety and style. In the man's part, only his lead indication is altered; on the first triple-time step, he moves the woman to a tuck position by turning her toward his right side with the fingers of his right hand. On the second triple-time step, he leads her into the underarm turn. (Another version of the tuck turn is to omit the underarm turn and simply release the woman's hands on her turn and rejoin the same hands after her unassisted pivot as she moves to full open position.) The tuck position is in the opposite direction of the turn to assist in gaining momentum for the rotation.

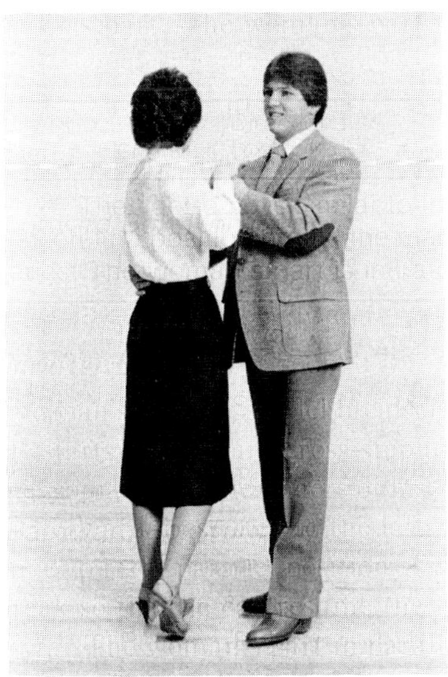

Figure 5.3. Tuck position

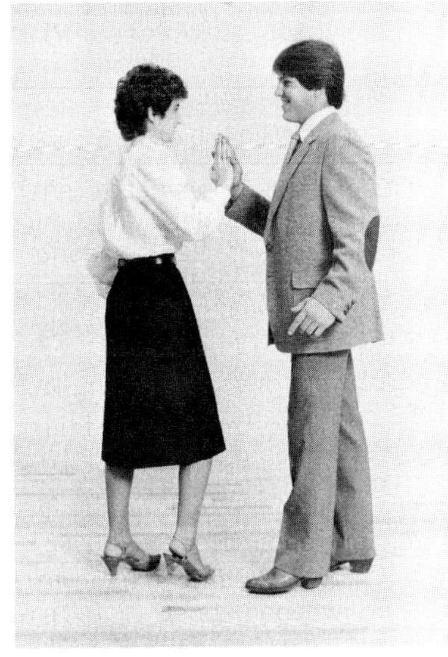

Figure 5.4. Hand-push tuck turn

Hand-Push Tuck Turn

As the name implies, this tuck turn is given impetus by a push of the joined hands. Both dancers use the heel of the hand and a tight, resistful arm during the pushing action which initiates the turn. (Another version is to face the partner directly, right palms touching. After the turn, man uses left hand for the "get-out.")

Interchanges and Equivalents

The adept swing dancer should be capable of improvisation and quick changes within the various components of the basic steps. These interchanges can be incorporated only after the dancer has an understanding of the rhythm and style of each of the basic steps and the differences between them.

Step-Pattern	Timing	Cue	Equivalents
Single-time	S	Step or Step-hit	Step-dip (bend knees) or step-bend or step-stomp (no wt-ct 2)
Double-time	q q	Touch-step or Dig-step	Kick-step or tuck-spin or stomp-step (no wt chg on ct 1)
Triple-time	q & q	Step-tog-step	Coaster step (ct 1—bwd, ct &—bwd, ct 2—fwd) or Turn–2–3
Break Step	q q	Rock-step	Hitch-kick (ct 1—kick fwd no wt, ct &—bwd rock, ct 2—fwd step) or walk, walk (fwd, fwd—can also incorporate swivels on ball of ft)

Another example of interchanges and equivalents is to combine two of the basic rhythms, such as double-time and triple-time. This will produce a medium-slow tempo and can change the style of the step pattern. Since each of the basic rhythms takes the same number of counts, they are all interchangeable; however, the combination of single-time with either of the other two basic rhythms may feel awkward when put to music and is not encouraged.

The West Coast swing basic step exemplifies this affirmation. It mixes double-time and triple-time rhythms with the break step and employs an equivalent for each.

West Coast Swing Basic Step

Starting Position—Join hands, man's L, woman's R, face partner directly

Step-Pattern	Directional Cue	Count	Timing Cue	Foot (Man)	Foot (Lady)	Comments
Double-time	IP	1, 2	q,q	L, L	R, R	"Kick" using ct 1 to lift foot fwd with no wt chg. Ct 2 is "step" and chg wt.
Triple-time	IP	3 & 4	q & q	R,L,R	L,R,L	"Coast-er-step" or "back, back, fwd" or "flat, ball, flat."
Break step	IP	5,6	q,q	L, R	R, L	"Walk, walk." Both dancers can walk fwd twd partner, or the man can walk bwd as the woman moves fwd. The man can also lead a swivel by moving his bent L arm (and her resistful R arm) to his L and then across in frt to his R; she swivels on the ball of each ft by turning toes out and heel in as wt is changed to other ft.

Note: The basic step can be altered by placing the break step first and would thus be cued as: "walk, walk, kick-step, coaster-step." Variations such as underarm turns, tuck turns and others are incorporated into this slower, western-style of swing. Its tempo can be danced to country-western, blues or other relaxed swing music.

Eight Count Swing Rhythms

A basic step that has eight counts will require measures of music that are even in number and thus will coincide perfectly with most swing music. These also add variety to the dancer's repetoire of swing step patterns.

Lindy Basic

Starting Position: Couple faces opp. dir. in swing hand-hold (R sd hips tog.)

Step-Pattern	Directional Cue	Count	Timing Cue	Foot (Man)	Foot (Lady)	Comments
Triple-Time	CW	1 & 2	q & q	L,R,L	R,L,R	Turning half basic cued as "turn–2–3."
Step, Step	CW	3,4	q,q	R,L	L,R	Continue turning on these two fwd walking steps, "walk, walk." Styling—shift hip to sd after each step.
Triple-Time	IP	5 & 6	q & q	R,L,R	L,R,L	Stop the turn, break apart to full open pos. and complete a coaster step. Cued as "back, back, fwd."
Break Step	CW	7,8	q,q	L,R	R,L	Continue walking fwd twd partner so as to repeat process. "Walk, walk."

Note: The rhythm and step pattern should be attempted in place first without the turning action. This is cued as "1-2-3, walk, walk, 1-2-3, walk, walk." Here, lindy basic is similar to triple-time basic, with the exception of adding two steps in between the two triples. This will require slower music. There are variations of the lindy basic which involve other turns and whips.

Shag Basic
Starting Position: Semiopen Position

Step-Pattern	Directional Cue	Count	Timing Cue	Foot (Man)	Foot (Lady)	Comments
Triple-Time	IP	1 & 2	q & q	L,R,L	R,L,R	Cue words: "tri-ple time." Other alternatives are single-time and double-time.
Kick	Fwd	3	q	R	L	"Kick" ft fwd with wt on other ft. Kick away from partner.
Hop	IP	4	q	L	R	"Hop" on ft with no wt chg.
Step	IP	5	q	R	L	"Step" with wt on ft
Stomp	IP	6	q	L	R	"Stomp" ft to floor with no wt chg. (Keep wt. back on supporting leg). Lift free foot up next.
Step	IP	7	q	L	R	"Rock" fwd to chg wt to same ft that stomped.

Step-Pattern	Directional Cue	Count	Timing Cue	Foot (Man)	Foot (Lady)	Comments
Step	IP	8	q	R	L	"Step" bwd with wt chg.

Note: The shag is compatible with very fast swing music, but it should be practiced slowly at first. It can incorporate a ¼ or ½ turn on the hop (ct 4) by turning twd partner and then resuming orig. pos. by again turning twd partner on the "rock-step" (ct 7–8). There are many variations to shag basic. When well-executed, shag is guaranteed to draw attention on the dance floor.

Suggested Sequence:

4 single-time basics

4 double-time basics

4 triple-time basics (the last two can be turning basics)

2 throw-out variations

2 underarm turn (with exchange) variations (tucks can be added)

3 hand-push tuck turns

4 West Coast swing basics

3 lindy basic turns

4 shag basics

Suggested Musical Selections:

"Kansas City," Wilbert Harrison, MCA Records, D-2524.

"Shop Around," Captain & Tennille, A&M Forget Me Nots, 8600-S.

"Billie Jean," Michael Jackson, Mijac Music (BMI), Warner Tamerlane (BMI).

polka and similar regional dances

6

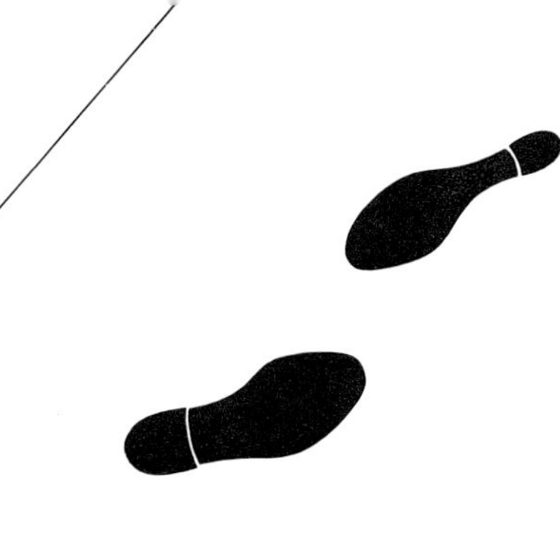

The polka was an innovation of a Czech servant girl, Anna Chadimova, before it was taken to Prague, the capital of Bohemia (a province of Czechoslovakia), in the early 1800s. The word polka was derived from the Czech term "pulka," meaning half, which refers to the half step used in the dance. In 1844, one Paris newspaper reported that the Polka embraced in its qualities the intimacy of the waltz with the vivacity of the Irish jig. It was met with opposition at first, named irreligious and immoral, almost everywhere it was introduced. The United States was no exception when it became the rage in the latter half of the nineteenth century. However, its popularity could not be restrained, and the polka endured. It is usually considered to be a folk dance form, but most social dance classes also want to learn its step patterns. The Polish polka or "hot" polka has a double hop and is more difficult to learn. A unique combination of polka with swing variations is an advanced form of creativity for even more enjoyment. Both swing and polka use a clockwise rotational triple-time step and therefore can be inter-related to encourage faster learning for everyone.

Timing

Most polka music is written in $\frac{2}{4}$ or cut-time. It can be performed either fast or medium fast and its timing is cued "and quick 'n quick" or "and 1 'n 2". The accent should be on the "and." Some ethnic dancers add other rhythmic patterns for variety.

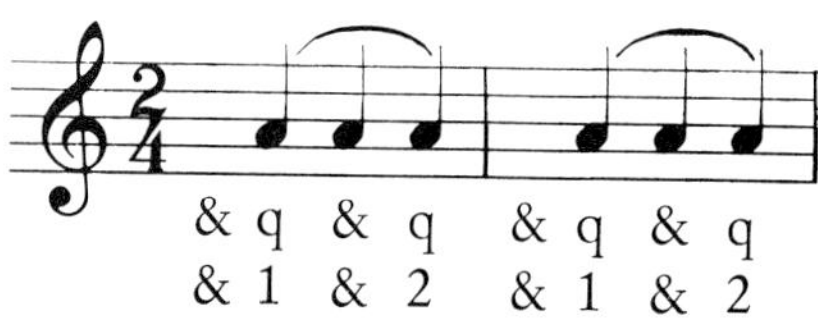

Figure 6.1. Polka rhythmic pattern

Styling

The polka is a bright and energetic dance in which enthusiasm becomes contagious. Overzealous participants should be reminded that the traveling rotational patterns must be performed in moderation to ensure the safety of other class members. The polka is not a wild dance; it has proper styling. The basic step is simply a hop and a triple-time step, alternating from side to side. A swaying motion is incorporated by looking and leaning in the direction of travel. On the hop, the foot is lifted at a height between the ankle and the knee and diagonally to the rear. The closed-couple dance position is modified so that the dancers stand slightly apart, allowing for the hopping action. Some dancers prefer folk dance positions such as the promenade position, where they stand side-by-side facing direction of dance (CCW), or the shoulder-waist position, where they face each other at arm's length.

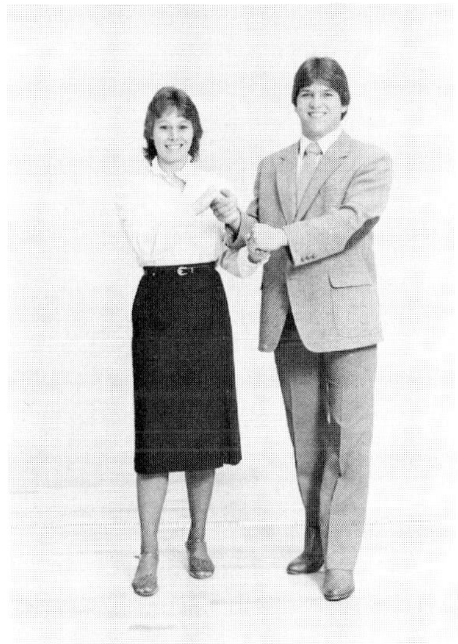

Figure 6.2. Promenade position

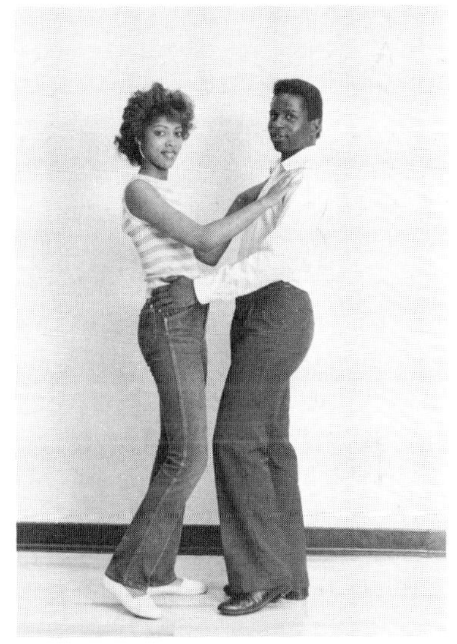

Figure 6.3. Shoulder-waist position

Basic Step

(Man faces direction of dance)

Step	Foot	Directional Cue	Count	Timing Cue	Comments
First Half-Basic (Man performs this part first)					
1	R	IP	&	&	L ft is unweighted, hop on R ft (Cue—"Hop")
2	L	Sd	1	q	"Flat" (A triple-time step is taken toward the ctr of CCW circle)

Step	Foot	Directional Cue	Count	Timing Cue	Comments
3	R	Tog	&	&	"Ball"
4	L	Sd	2	q	"Flat"

Second Half-Basic (Woman performs this part first)

Step	Foot	Directional Cue	Count	Timing Cue	Comments
5	L	IP	&	&	R ft is unweighted, hop on L ft (Cue—"hop")
6	R	Sd	1	q	"Flat" (A triple-time step is taken toward the outside wall)
7	L	Tog	&	&	"Ball"
8	R	Sd	2	q	"Flat"

Note: Woman's part is in natural opposition to the man's. On the first half-basic, the couple moves toward the center of the circle. On the second half-basic, they move away from the center of the circle.

Turning Basic

(Man faces direction of dance)

Step	Foot	Directional Cue	Count	Timing Cue	Comments

First Half-Basic

Step	Foot	Directional Cue	Count	Timing Cue	Comments
1	R	CW	&	&	¼CW turn so as to mnvr to face outside wall on the hop. After first time, ½ turn is taken.
2	L	Sd	1	q	(A triple-time step is taken to the L toward direction of dance)
3	R	Tog	&	&	
4	L	Sd	2	q	

Second Half-Basic

Step	Foot	Directional Cue	Count	Timing Cue	Comments
5	L	CW	&	&	½CW turn on the hop
6	R	Sd	1	q	(A triple-time step is taken to the R toward direction of dance)
7	L	Tog	&	&	
8	R	Sd	2	q	

Note: Woman's part is in natural opposition to the man's. The triple-time step is always taken toward direction of dance. The hop serves as the tool for turning and manuevering. (Cue: "turn, triple-time-step.")

Forward Basic

(Both parts face direction of dance in promenade position). The basic step can also be performed in a forward direction.

Step	Foot	Directional Cue	Count	Timing Cue	Comments
First Half-Basic					
1	R	IP	&	&	"Hop"
2	L	Fwd	1	q	"Flat" (A triple-time step is taken fwd. It is also called a two-step, even though three steps are taken—in the ct of 2)
3	R	Tog	&	&	"Ball" This is a half-step—the toes of the back ft meet the instep of the fwd ft.
4	L	Fwd	2	q	"Flat"
Second Half-Basic					
5	L	IP	&	&	"Hop"
6	R	Fwd	1	q	"Flat" (This time the triple-time step starts with the R ft—in alternation)
7	L	Tog	&	&	"Ball" (Half-step)
8	R	Fwd	2	q	"Flat"

Note: Woman again performs the second half-basic while man performs the first half-basic. *Variation:* The heel-and-toe polka could be added to the forward basic. The man places his left heel diagonally to his left for counts "and-one" (no weight change); then he crosses his left foot in front of the right foot (no weight change) to place the toes of his left foot to the floor for "and-two" counts. The first half-basic is then performed. The same sequence is repeated to the right. The woman's part can be either in natural opposition to the man's or the same as the man's, whichever is preferred.

Suggested Sequence:

4 heel-and-toe polka variations

8 forward basics

8 turning basics

Suggested Musical Selections:

"Beer Barrel Polka," Hoctor, #601.

"Heel and Toe Polka," MacGregor Records, #5003 (Box 644, Pumona, CA 91769).

SIMILAR REGIONAL DANCES

There are other regional dances that are similar to the polka and can be included in this unit. Country-western attire and music are encouraged.

Schottische

The word "schottische" means literally "Scottish," thus having its origins in Scotland. Timing is the primary difference between the polka and the schottische. The time signature is $\frac{2}{4}$ for the polka and $\frac{4}{4}$ for the schottische. Also, the hop is performed on count one in the Polka, but not until count four in the schottische. The cue words for the schottische are: "1–2–3–hop"—"1–2–3–4"— so that one full count is allowed for each step. The sequence alternates from one side to the other, either laterally or forward, and then a series of four step-hops are added. The man's part is cued as: "L,R,L, hop—R,L,R,hop—L, hop, R, hop, L, hop, R, hop." The woman's part is in opposition, and she can perform an underarm turn on the step-hops. Promenade position is used.

Two-Step

Another name for the "two-step" is the triple-time step, which is the basic component of the polka. It has also been used as the basic step of country-western style of dance. The "hop" in the polka is replaced by a soft shuffle, and often another one-count walking step is added for variety of rhythm and step-pattern. The partners usually face each other so that the man can travel forward in direction of dance and the woman is in natural opposition. They can assume basic closed-dance position or a modification called a Texas-style hold in which the woman hooks the thumb of her L hand in the belt loop on his R side, and the man places his R hand on her L shoulder. Variations include a turning basic in CW direction and underarm turns. Promenade position can also be used. Cue words are: "brush, flat, ball, flat."

Note: The Texas two-step may also be taught as a combined form of the magic step in fox-trot and single-time swing (S,S,q,q). The Texas-style hold is incorporated. The man starts with his L ft, the woman starts with her R ft. The cue words are:

```
      1     2      3     4      5     6
"Side-touch,  Side-touch,  walk, walk."
     L-R   ,   R-L   ,   L,   R
```

The man usually travels fwd on the walking steps.

Cotton-Eyed Joe

This dance is traditionally performed to a duple-rhythm fiddle hoedown of the same name. It has been perpetuated over many generations and has become public domain. It is usually included in country-western dance basics. The promenade position is used with a partner, but the dance can also be performed in a long line of adjacent dancers who place their arms around the waist (or shoulders) of the person beside them. Everyone uses the same foot in unison throughout the dance. A simple version of this basic routine is: Part 1—R ft is unweighted and crosses in front of L leg just below the knee for count one; then R leg kicks forward about one foot high for count two. Cue words are: "hook, kick." A triple-time step, starting with the R foot, R-L-R, follows for counts three and four. This triple-time step can be performed in place, forward, sideward or as a coaster step. The sequence is then repeated for four counts, starting with the L foot. The entire sequence is repeated for a total of 16 counts. Part 2 consists of eight two-steps forward, starting with the R foot, for a total of 16 counts. Repeat Part 1 and Part 2. Music: Asylum Records #E–46640-B. "The Unstrung Heroes— Cotton-Eyed Joe."

latin rhythm dances

The rhythm dances, which were native to the Latin-American countries, are known as the Latin rhythm dances. Their heritage is of African and Spanish influence primarily. They are "spot dances," not traveling dances, and can be performed in relatively small areas of space. They were developed during the first half of the twentieth century and are considered to be among the more recent of the traditional ballroom dances.

The music of the Latin rhythm dances has a distinctive sound because of the use of these instruments: the maracas, which are dried gourds filled with buckshot and shook in time with the music; the bongo drums, which consist of two small joined drums that are placed between the knees and beaten with the bare hands; and the claves, which are made of two pieces of hard wood about 6×1 inches in size and are struck together to create a sharp and reverberating sound. Latin music remains popular with many recording stars and is easy to obtain for the Latin rhythm dance enthusiast.

The Latin hold is similar to the basic closed-couple dance position, but the elbows are elevated more. This is especially true in the Cuban dances.

The Latin rhythm dances to be included are the samba (a bouncy rotational dance), the merengue (a simple, preparatory dance for Cuban motion), and the Cuban dances (the mambo, cha-cha and rumba).

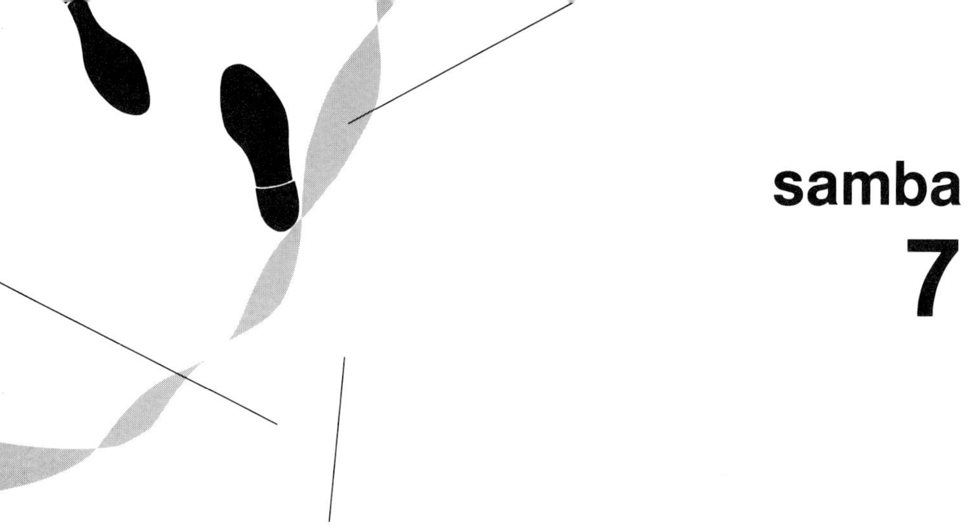

samba
7

Samba is the national dance of Brazil. Its first form to be seen abroad was the maxixe, which was an exhibition dance of the early 1900s. It reappeared in the late 1930s as the samba. The "Brazilian Bombshell," Carmen Miranda (an American movie star), helped to popularize the samba, and the dance reached its peak in the 1950s. Another form of the samba, combined with a twist of the hips on each beat, was called the bossa nova and was popular for a short time in the 1960s. Of all the Latin rhythm dances, the samba is probably the most light-hearted and festive.

Timing

Samba music is played in $\frac{2}{4}$ time and is recognized by its lilting, bouncy rhythm.

The tempo can be either slow or fast, but the latter is usually preferred. For each measure of two beats there are three weight changes, and the starting foot alternates. The cues are "quick-and-quick" or "1 or 2."

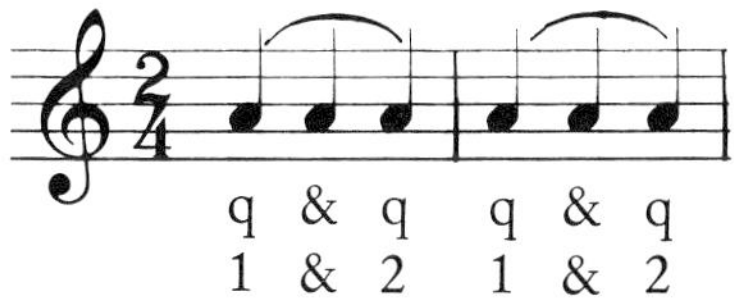

Figure 7.1. Samba rhythmic pattern

Styling

Samba, like the other Latin rhythm dances, emphasizes hip-action. The pelvis is moved forward and backward and acts as a hinge between the upper and lower body parts. The feet initiate the direction of movement to allow a controlled springing action involving the ball of the foot, the relaxed ankle and the flexed knee. The upper body (above the diaphragm area) remains stationary as the hips and feet swing forward and backward in rhythm to the music. Various dance positions may be used in samba, but the basic closed Latin dance position is most common.

Basic Step

The box step is the basic step of the samba. We previously learned the four-count box step in fox-trot and the three-count box step in waltz; now, a two-count box step will be presented in samba. It would be helpful to review a few step patterns of the waltz so as to interrelate them to the samba. The "rise and fall" styling of the waltz is different from that of the samba. To learn the samba motion, start with your feet together in first parallel foot position and try, on count "and," rising on the toes with the legs straight. Then, on count "one," bend the knees. Repeat the action for counts "and," "two." Practice first without the music until the movement feels natural. Then attempt to keep time with the music. If this is successful, add the samba motion to the preliminary footwork, which is the same as the waltz balance (forward and backward). Incorporating the two-count rhythm, the man rises up on his toes, preparing to step forward with his left foot for count "and." As he places his weight on his left foot, he bends the knees for count "one." His right foot steps forward to a position beside the left—rise on toes for count "and." His left foot steps in place—bend knees for count "two." Repeat the same bouncing action, starting with the right foot for a backward balance. Remember that on every "and" count there is a toe rise with knees straight and on every "one" or "two" the knees are bent.

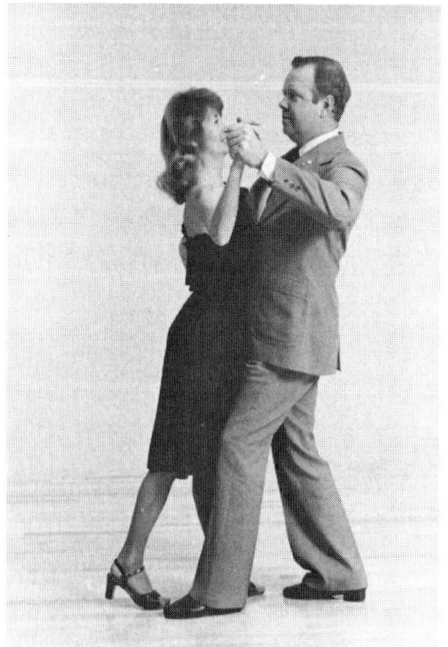

Figure 7.2. Samba motion

Samba Box Step

(Man's part—the woman's part is in natural opposition)

Step	Foot	Directional Cue	Count	Timing Cue	Comments
Forward Half Box					
1	L	IP	&	&	Rise on toes, brush L ft fwd as hips push fwd
2	L	Fwd	1	q	Bend knees, wt on L ft
3	R	Sd	&	&	Rise on toes, legs str
4	L	Tog	2	q	Bend knees
Backward Half Box					
1	R	IP	&	&	Rise on toes, brush R ft bwd as hips pull bwd
2	R	Bwd	1	q	Bend knees, wt on R ft
3	L	Sd	&	&	Rise on toes, legs str
4	R	Tog	2	q	Bend knees

Note: The man starts with the forward half box and the woman starts with the backward half box. The parts are then alternated.

Turn

Left Box Turn

(Man's part—the woman's part is in natural opposition)

Step	Foot	Directional Cue	Count	Timing Cue	Comments
Forward Box Turn (¼)					
1	L	IP	&	&	Rise on toes, hips push fwd, L ft starts fwd arc-shaped CCW turn
2	L	Fwd	1	q	Bend knees, wt on L ft (facing ¼ to the L)
3	R	Sd	&	&	Directly to the R sd. Rise on toes, legs str
4	L	Tog	2	q	Bend knees
Backward Box Turn (¼)					
1	R	IP	&	&	Rise on toes, hips push bwd, R ft starts bwd ¼ CCW turn
2	R	Bwd	1	q	Bend knees, wt on R ft (facing the opp. wall from orig. dir.)
3	L	Sd	&	&	Directly to L sd. Rise on toes.
4	R	Tog	2	q	Bend knees

Note: Repeat to complete full turn. The woman begins with the backward box turn.

Variations

Chasse

(Man's part—the woman's part is in natural opposition)

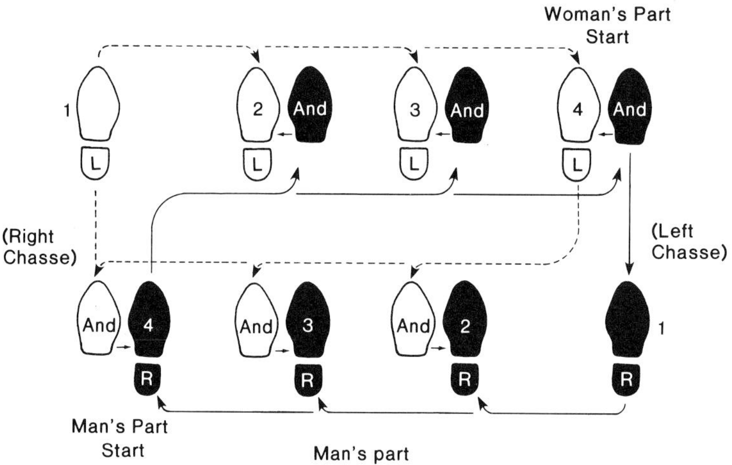

Figure 7.3. Chassé step

Step	Foot	Directional Cue	Count	Timing Cue	Comments
Right Chasse					
1	L	IP	&	&	Rise on toes, hips push fwd and brush L ft fwd
2	L	Fwd	1	q	Bend knees, wt on L ft
3	R	Sd	&	&	Directly to R sd. Rise on toes.
4	L	Tog	2	q	Bend knees
5	R	Sd	&	&	Directly to R sd. Rise on toes.
6	L	Tog	3	q	Bend knees
7	R	Sd	&	&	Directly to R sd. Rise on toes.
8	L	Tog	4	q	Bend knees
Left Chasse					
1	R	IP	&	&	Rise on toes, hips push bwd and brush R ft bwd
2	R	Bwd	1	q	Bend knees, wt on R ft
3	L	Sd	&	&	Directly to L sd. Rise on toes.
4	R	Tog	2	q	Bend knees
5	L	Sd	&	&	Directly to L sd. Rise on toes.

Step	Foot	Directional Cue	Count	Timing Cue	Comments
6	R	Tog	3	q	Bend knees
7	L	Sd	&	&	Directly to L sd. Rise on toes.
8	R	Tog	4	q	Bend knees

Note: The woman begins with the left chassé and then completes the right chassé.

Copacabana Step

(Man's part—woman starts with the Right Copa)

The "copa" progresses forward in conversation position. Start in closed-couple dance position first.

Step	Foot	Directional Cue	Count	Timing Cue	Comments
Left Copa					
1	L	IP	&	&	Turn the woman to conversation pos. Rise on toes, hips push fwd and brush L ft fwd. Tip body sl bwd.
2	L	Fwd	1	q	Bend knees, wt on L ft
3	R	Bwd	&	&	Rise on toes, legs str, wt on R ft. Tip body sl fwd. "Rock"—leave L ft fwd.
4	L	IP	2	q	Bend knees, wt on L ft. "Step"
Right Copa					
1	R	IP	&	&	Rise on toes, hips push fwd and brush R ft fwd. Tip body sl bwd.
2	R	Fwd	3	q	Bend knees, wt on R ft
3	L	Bwd	&	&	Rise on toes, legs str, wt on L ft.
4	R	IP	4	q	Bend knees, wt on R ft

Note: This step pattern can also be performed in open position. It allows more freedom of movement so that the body can turn slightly in the same direction as the working foot and the outside hands can make contact when the dancers turn alternately toward each other. Repeat the step pattern as desired.

The "copa" can also be performed in the reverse direction if the open position is used. The last right copa of the series serves as the transition step by the couple moving toward each other and completing one half turn to face the opposite direction. They change arms and are ready to proceed with a left copa toward the partner, and the series is repeated. The "get-out" is to use the transition step on a left copa toward the partner and assume closed-couple dance position.

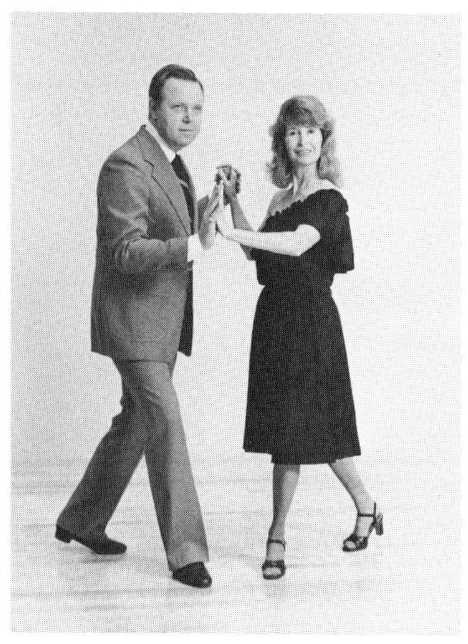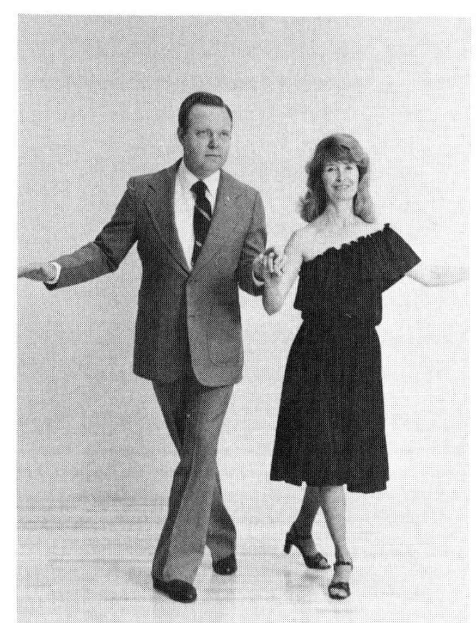

Figure 7.4. Copacabana

Suggested Sequence:

2 box steps (complete)
1 left box turn (complete)
2 chassé variations (complete)
2 copacabana steps (forward and reverse)

Suggested Musical Selections:

"Copacabana," vocalist—Barry Manilow, Flashback Records, Arista Records, Inc., FLB 101.
"Tico Tico," Hoctor, #611.
"Anna," Hoctor, #1615.
"Brazil," Hoctor, #603.

merengue

8

The merengue (pronounced ma-reng-gay) is the national dance of Haiti, which is near the Dominican Republic. The Dominican version became popular in the United States in the mid–1950s. Supposedly, its traditional "limp step" of hip and knee action was first used by a lame Dominican general who refused to give up dancing at a party, so his guests imitated his movements respectfully. As the dance was refined, it was done either in a suave, sophisticated manner or a light, breezy fashion. Of the Latin rhythm dances, it is one of the easiest to learn.

Timing

Merengue music has a subtle syncopation in that the second of its two counts is stressed more than the first. It is similar to samba music but has a stronger beat and is often less melodic. Timing cues are "quick, quick," or "1, 2." The tempo is $\frac{2}{4}$ with a bright, staccato sound.

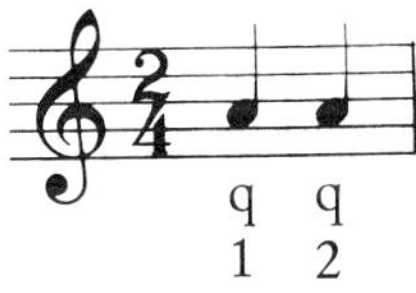

Figure 8.1. Merengue rhythmic pattern

Styling

The merengue is associated with "lame-duck styling," which is used on count one of each measure. It is similar to Cuban motion hip swing, but a slight limp is used. The basic closed Latin dance position is necessary, and the shoulders can remain level or dip on the lame side, whichever method is preferred. Footwork involves the ball to a flat foot on each step, is similar to a chassé performed slowly, and is cued "apart, together." Most step patterns are performed for eight counts (or four basics).

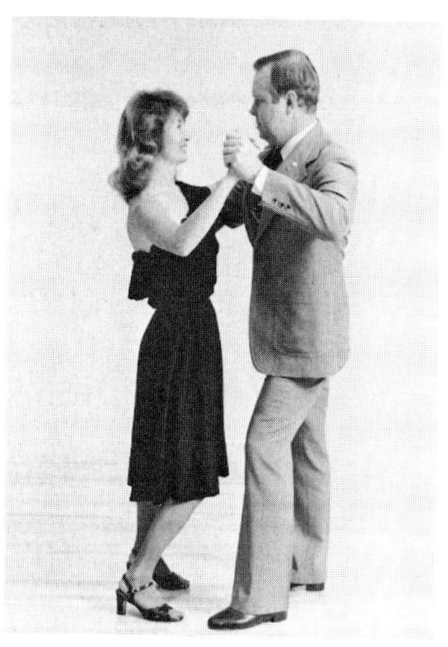

Figure 8.2. Lame duck

Basic Steps

The merengue basic step can be performed sideward, forward and backward. "Lame-duck styling" is incorporated on odd-numbered counts.

Step	Foot	Directional Cue	Count	Timing Cue	Comments
Man's Part					
Side Basic					
1	L	Sd	1	q	Small step to L sd (in 2nd pos.) with a limp
2	R	Tog	2	q	Body erect
Forward Basic					
1	L	Fwd	1	q	Small step fwd (in 4th pos.) with a limp
2	R	Tog	2	q	Body erect. To travel, allow the R ft to pass the L ft
Backward Basic					
1	L	Bwd	1	q	Small step bwd with a limp
2	R	Tog	2	q	Body erect. To travel, allow the R ft to pass the L ft
Box Step					
Forward Half Box					
1	L	Fwd	1	q	Small step fwd with a limp
2	R	IP	2	q	Body straightens, but leave L ft fwd

Step	Foot	Directional Cue	Count	Timing Cue	Comments
		Backward Half Box			
1	L	Bwd	1	q	Bring L ft bwd with a limp
2	R	IP	2	q	Body straightens, R ft stays in place throughout sequence

Combinations

The basic steps can be combined in different ways:

1. A series of one forward basic and one side basic
2. A series of one backward basic and one side basic
3. Four side basics and two box steps

Step	Foot	Directional Cue	Count	Timing Cue	Comments
Woman's Part					
Side Basic					
1	R	Sd	1	q	Small step to R sd with a limp
2	L	Tog	2	q	Body erect
Forward Basic					
1	R	Bwd	1	q	Small step bwd with a limp
2	L	Tog	2	q	Body erect. To travel, allow the L ft to pass the R ft.
Backward Basic					
1	R	Fwd	1	q	Small step fwd with a limp
2	L	Tog	2	q	Body erect. To travel, allow the L ft to pass the R ft.
Box Step					
		Forward Half Box			
1	R	Bwd	1	q	Small step bwd with a limp
2	L	IP	2	q	Body straightens, but leave R ft bwd
		Backward Half Box			
1	R	Fwd	1	q	Bring R ft fwd with a limp
2	L	IP	2	q	Body straightens; L ft stays in place throughout sequence

Turns
Left Box Turn

Step	Foot	Directional Cue	Count	Timing Cue	Comments
Man's Part					
Forward Half Box (¼)					
1	L	Fwd	1	q	Arc-shaped ¼ CCW turn with a limp, ft in 4th pos. (R ft stays in place)
2	R	Tog	2	q	Body erect
Backward Half Box (¼)					
1	L	Bwd	1	q	Turn 1 ft ¼CCW first (limp), ft in 3rd pos. (R ft stays in place)
2	R	Tog	2	q	Body erect
Woman's Part					
Forward Half Box (¼)					
1	R	Bwd	1	q	Turn R ft ¼ CCW first (limp), ft form a "T." (L ft stays in place)
2	L	Tog	2	q	Body erect, ft parallel.
Backward Half Box (¼)					
1	R	Fwd	1	q	¼ CCW turn with a limp
2	L	Tog	2	q	Body erect, ft parallel

Note: Keep circumference of turn small. Allow the pos. of the limp to aid the turn.

Underarm Turn

The man's part of the underarm turn is to lead the woman under the arch formed by his left arm and her right arm. He lightly pushes her with his right hand in the desired direction as he performs the side basic.

The woman walks forward as she assumes arch position and turns in a clockwise circle under the man's arm. The couple then resumes the basic closed-couple dance position.

Circle Turn

In circle turns, the man travels with the forward basic to his left in a counter-clockwise circle (either small or large as preferred). The length of the step differs—take long steps on odd-numbered steps (with "lame duck styling") and take short steps on even-numbered steps. The woman's part is in natural opposition to the man's.

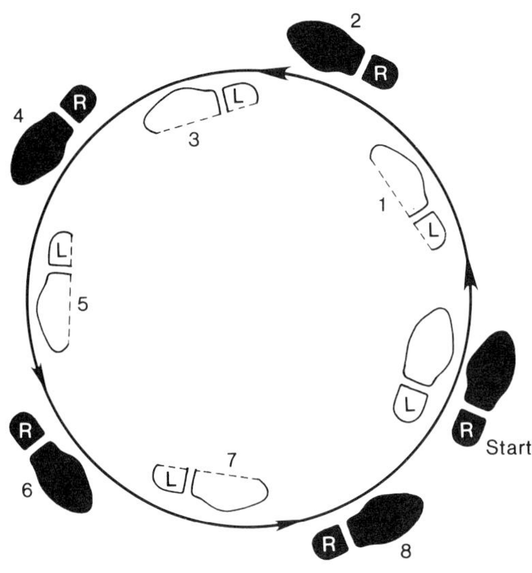

Figure 8.3. Circle turn

Suggested Sequence: (start with man facing outside wall and woman facing in)

8 side basics

4 box steps (complete)

4 forward basics

4 backward basics

2 left box turns (complete)

2 circle turns

Suggested Musical Selections:

"Calypso Breakdown," Ralph MacDonald, Original Movie Soundtrack of Saturday Night Fever, RSO Records, Inc.

"Por Un Pelito," Hoctor, #680.

"El Negrito," Hoctor, #680.

"Merengue No. 28," Hoctor, #625.

"Compadre Piatro," Hoctor, #625.

"I Ain't Down Yet," Dance Along Records, #P-6080.

the cuban dances

The Latin rhythm dances that originated in Cuba are the cha-cha, mambo and rumba. They make up the Cuban system (with the exception of a slow rumba exhibition dance called the bolero), and they are characterized by Cuban motion styling. This should be introduced first so that it can later be incorporated into the step patterns of the Cuban dances. The student should be directed to stand in proper posture facing a full-length mirror (if available), akimbo or hands on hips. Try pushing with the right hand so that the right hip sways laterally to the left side. The movement should be soft, slight and well-controlled. The upper torso remains stationary throughout. The left leg should straighten and accept the body weight as the right knee bends and is freed of body weight. Try the same motion to the opposite side so that the hips move, softly swaying, from side to side. Repeat several times before attempting to walk with the motion. (The man's hip action should be barely noticeable compared to the woman's.) As one leg bends, the other straightens and accepts the body weight. In order to incorporate the walk, continue with the right knee bent and weight-free. Students are ready to take a short step in the intended direction, with the weight transferring first through the ball to the heel of the right foot. When students step in a flat-footed manner, the hips then shift to the right naturally, but with assistance of a little push of the left hand for the present. As the right leg assumes the body weight, the left foot is ready to take a step. The process continues with a hip shift to the opposite side, unweighting first before taking each step. As the students progress, they should try to move in all four directions, move the hands to the "W-position," move to the beat of Latin music and then try to coordinate the Cuban motion walk with partners in dance position. A couple's movements should be natural in response to the rhythm and melody of the music.

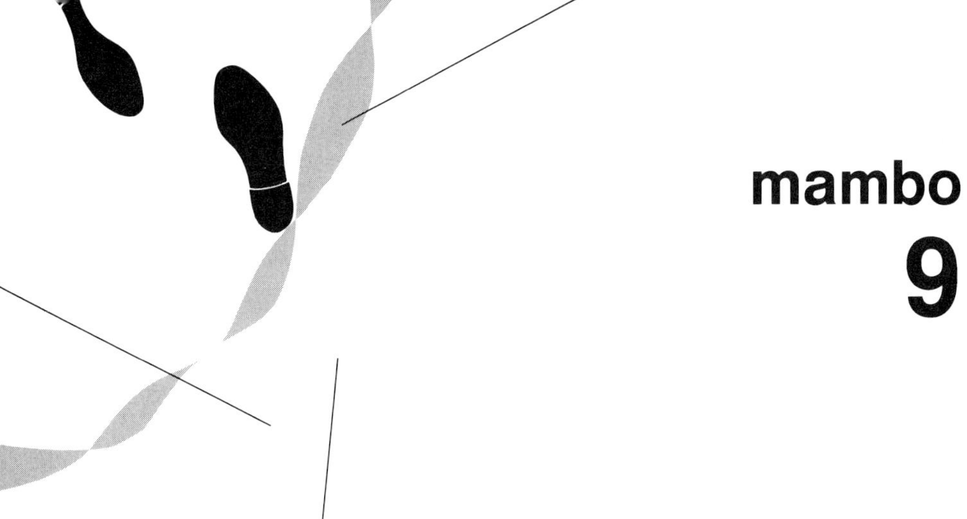

mambo
9

The name mambo was derived from an African appellation for a voodoo cult priestess. It was developed around 1950 as the syncopated swing music influenced the already present rumba beat, and it became a combination of the two. Many of the step patterns in both mambo and cha-cha can be interchanged because of their similarities. Therefore, cross-references will be used in this text between the two dances.

Timing

The primary difference found in mambo and cha-cha is their rhythm. Mambo has a distinctive offbeat $\frac{4}{4}$ rhythm in which the counts of two and four are accented. Like swing, it can be done in single-time (fast), double-time (medium) and triple-time (slow). The most common mambo basic step is the single-time version, and therefore mambo is usually considered to be a faster dance rhythm than cha-cha.

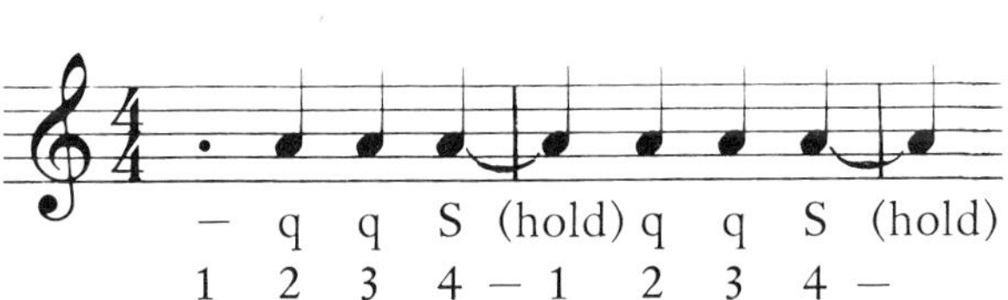

Figure 9.1. Mambo rhythmic pattern

Styling

Although the use of Cuban motion is the most predominant styling technique of
the Cuban dances, the mambo is also known for its use of free interpretation or
creative step patterns by its more proficient dancers. The basic positions are the
closed Latin dance position, the one-hand open position and the shine position.

Most variations in mambo (and cha-cha) are preceded and followed by the
basic step. The variation must not disturb the timing or the logical arrangement
of the forward and backward half-basics. Most variations will start to the man's
right and are usually performed in a series of three.

Mambo Basic Step

(Man's part—the woman's part is in natural opposition).

Step	Foot	Directional Cue	Count	Timing Cue	Comments
Forward Break—To start with the forward half-basic, touch the left foot in place for count 1 (as a preliminary step)					
1	L	Fwd	2	q	Use small, flat steps
2	R	IP	3	q	
3	L	Tog	4–1	S	Hold for 2 cts and proceed to backward break (without preliminary step)
Backward Break—To start the series with a backward half-basic, step to left side with left foot for count 1 (as a preliminary step)					
1	R	Bwd	2	q	
2	L	IP	3	q	
3	R	Tog	4–1	S	Hold for 2 cts and continue a series of forward and backward breaks (without the preliminary step)

Note: The method of starting the series depends upon the preliminary step chosen.
Cuban motion styling is incorporated after the basic footwork is learned. (Option—
a progressive style of footwork can also be added on step 3, counts 4–1, by allowing the working foot to pass the supporting foot in a walking motion.)

Break Variations

Open Break

In the mambo (and cha-cha) basic steps, the forward break always incorporates
the left foot stepping forward, and the backward break (excluding the preliminary step) always incorporates the right foot stepping backward. The open break
changes this procedure on the man's part only. As the woman takes her backward

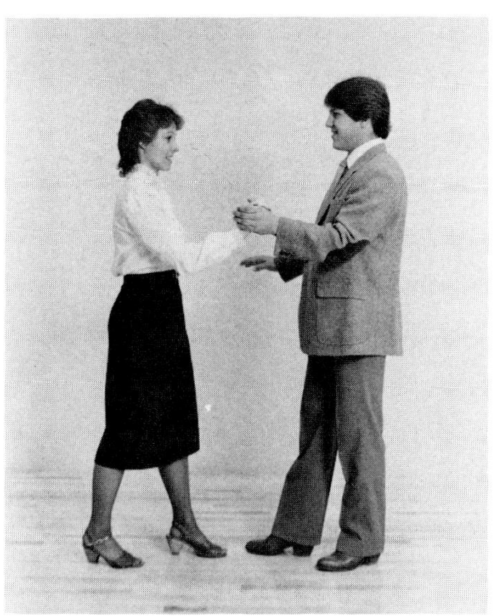

Figure 9.2. Open break

break, the man's left hand pushes and releases the woman's right hand to a one-hand open position as he breaks backward on his *left* foot. On the next step, his right foot moves forward toward the woman and they assume the original position. This step pattern replaces the man's forward break and results in three consecutive backward breaks for the man.

Crossover Breaks

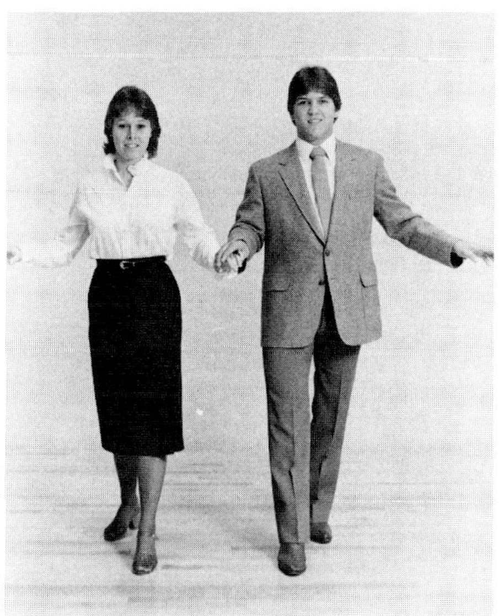

Figure 9.3. Crossover break

Step	Foot	Directional Cue	Count	Timing Cue	Comments
Right Crossover Break (must be preceded by a backward break)					
1	L	Fwd X	2	q	Cross L ft to face ¼ to the R. Lead—man's L hand takes woman's R hand at waist heighth, man's fingers on top of hers. Keep shoulders in a str line with partner's shoulders.
2	R	IP	3	q	R ft pivots in place to face twd partner
3	L	Tog	4–1	S	Hold for 2 cts
Left Crossover Break					
1	R	Fwd X	2	q	Cross R ft to face ¼ to the L. Lead—man's R hand takes woman's L hand as before. Ft in 4th pos.
2	L	IP	3	q	L ft pivots in place to face twd partner
3	R	Tog	4–1	S	Hold for 2 cts

Note: The man first leads a right crossover break while the woman performs a left crossover break. The parts are then reversed and continued as many times as desired. The step ends after the man's last left crossover break, and the forward break starts the basic step series again. Option—instead of the man's last left crossover break and the woman's last right crossover break, they both perform a walk-around turn as a "get-out." As a lead, the man pushes his right hand against her left hand, and both dancers turn away from each other after the cross to complete a small circle turn (man—CCW, woman—CW) on steps two and three. The man then resumes the forward break to start the basic step series again.

Fifth Position Breaks (Man leads the Right Fifth Position Break first)

Step	Foot	Directional Cue	Count	Timing Cue	Comments
Right Fifth Position Break (must be preceded by a forward break)					
1	R	Bwd	2	q	L ft stays in place, facing fwd, while rt moves bwd so that toes tch heel of L ft in 5th pos. Lead and couple's body positions are similar to that of the crossover breaks, except they are more tightly reigned.
2	L	IP	3	q	Wt chg
3	R	Tog	4–1	S	Hold 2 cts, facing partner

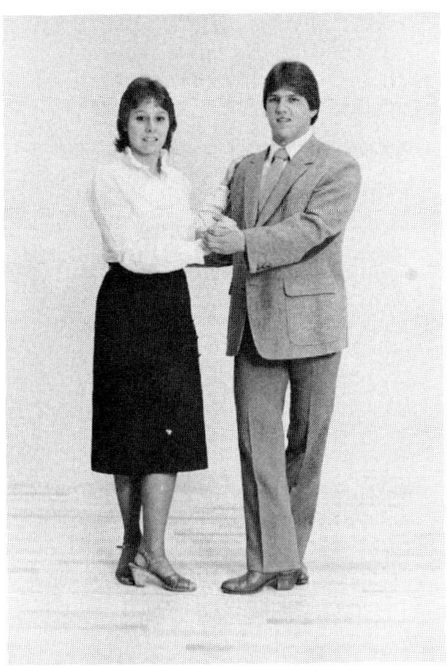

Figure 9.4. Fifth position breaks

Step	Foot	Directional Cue	Count	Timing Cue	Comments
Left Fifth Position Break					
1	L	Bwd	2	q	R ft stays in place, facing fwd, while L moves bwd so that toes tch heel of R ft in 5th pos. Lead to the L and same rules for body pos.
2	R	IP	3	q	Wt chg
3	L	Tog	4–1	S	Hold 2 cts, facing partner

Note: The "get-out" is similar to that of the crossover breaks, except that after the last left fifth position break, the man resumes the backward break of the basic step series. The woman's part is in natural opposition as in the crossover breaks.

Parallel Breaks

The man's part in parallel breaks is very similar to his part in the crossover breaks. He starts his forward cross-step to the right but steps diagonally forward to lead the woman with the fingers of his right hand to left parallel position. As he begins his forward cross-step to the left, he leads the woman with the fingers of his left hand to right parallel position. The series ends after the man's last left crossover break so that he can resume the forward break of the basic step.

Note: The woman's part in parallel breaks is very similar to her part in the fifth position breaks. As the man leads her to left parallel position, she steps backward with her right foot to face diagonally forward. In the right parallel position, she steps backward with her left foot to face diagonally forward. After this is repeated the desired number of times, the woman resumes the backward break of the basic step.

Suggested Sequence:

4 basic steps (complete)
4 open breaks
2 crossover breaks
2 fifth-position breaks

Suggested Musical Selections: (cha-cha music will slow the tempo)

"Perdido," Hoctor #622. (fast)
"Piel Canela," #622.

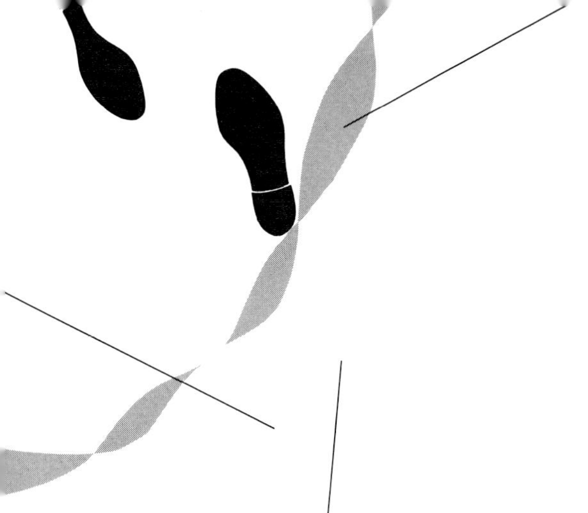

cha-cha
10

The name cha-cha has been derived from two possible sources: one indicates the sounds from the heelless slippers worn by the Cuban dancers performing the cha-cha; the other implies a similarity to the name of "chatch," which is the triple-time mambo step pattern from which the cha-cha was developed. It is a combination of mambo and swing and became popular during the 1950s. It is regarded as the most prevalent of all the Latin rhythm dances.

Timing

The cha-cha, like the mambo, is performed to $\frac{4}{4}$ music, but it is usually slower and has a more lively, staccato sound that accommodates the triple shuffles. It can be performed either on the offbeat or on the downbeat, but the offbeat is usually preferred. The music has a definite Latin flavor and is easy to obtain.

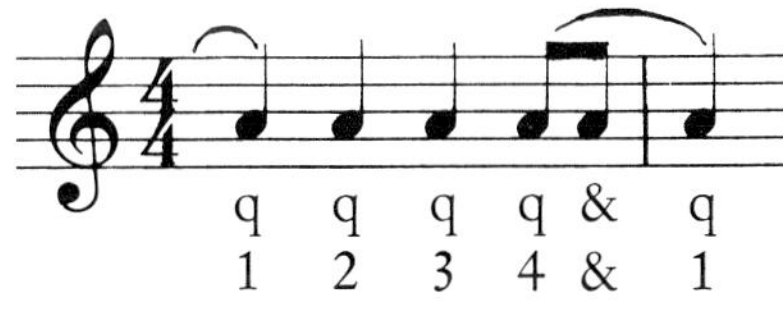

Figure 10.1. Cha-cha rhythmic pattern

Styling

Cha-cha styling is identical to mambo with these exceptions: the triple-time shuffle step is added, and it incorporates a smaller and a lighter foot pattern. A carefree, gay mood is reflected throughout this highly enjoyable dance.

Basic Step

The basic step for cha-cha is the same as the forward and backward breaks in mambo with one primary exception: the counts of 4–1 or the timing cue of "S" (slow) no longer consist of a "hold." Two "q's" (quicks) are added and are called "cha, cha." (The count of four is also called a "cha.")

Cha-Cha Basic

(Man's part—the woman's part is in natural opposition)

Step	Foot	Directional Cue	Count	Timing Cue	Comments
Forward Break—To start with the forward half-basic, touch the left foot in place for count 1 (as a preliminary step)					
1	L	Fwd	2	q	Use small, flat steps
2	R	IP	3	q	
3	L	Sd	4	q	Start a "triple-time" step to the L sd "Cha"
4	R	Tog	&	&	"Cha"
5	L	Sd	1	q	"Cha"
Backward Break—To start the series with a backward half-basic, step to left side with left foot for count 1 (as a preliminary step)					
1	R	Bwd	2	q	
2	L	IP	3	q	
3	R	Sd	4	q	Start a "triple-time" step to R sd, "Cha"
4	L	Tog	&	&	"Cha"
5	R	Sd	1	q	"Cha"

Note: The method of starting the series depends upon the preliminary step chosen. Cuban motion styling is incorporated after the basic footwork is learned. (Option— a progressive style of footwork can also be added on counts 4 & 1, or "Cha, Cha, Cha" by allowing the working foot to pass the supporting foot in a walking motion on each step.)

Break Variations

All of the breaks presented in mambo can be adapted to cha-cha by adding the triple-time step on the counts 4–1.

Turns

The turns in cha-cha (and mambo) require shine position, which is assumed by facing the partner directly, a comfortable distance apart, and releasing contact. The progressive style of footwork should be incorporated.

Half-Turn (Half Chase)

Step	Foot	Directional Cue	Count	Timing Cue	Comments
Forward Break Half-Turn—occurs in place of forward break in basic step					
1	L	Fwd	2	q	L ft steps fwd, R ft is behind in 4th parallel foot position
2	R	Fwd	3	q	½ pivot turn in place to face opp. dir. and immediately step fwd with R ft.
3	L	Fwd	4	q	Progressive style of footwork, walking fwd with feet passing. "Cha"
4	R	Fwd	&	&	"Cha"
5	L	Fwd	1	q	"Cha"
Backward Break Half-Turn—Occurs in place of backward break in basic step					
1	R	Fwd	2	q	R ft steps fwd, L ft is behind in 4th parallel foot pos., fcg reverse dir.
2	L	Fwd	3	q	½ pivot turn in place to face orig. dir. and immediately step fwd with L ft.
3	R	Fwd	4	q	Walk fwd for first "Cha"
4	L	Fwd	&	&	"Cha"
5	R	Fwd	1	q	"Cha"

Note: The man performs his forward break half-turn first as the lady performs her backward break of the basic step. Each half-turn therefore is in opposition, i.e., the man's backward break half-turn is complimented by the woman's forward break half-turn and vice-versa. (Option—to enhance the appearance of a chase step, the dancer in front is tapped on the turning shoulder by the dancer in the rear.) The "get-out" is to replace the man's forward break half-turn with the forward break of the basic step and the woman does likewise.

Full Turn (Full Chase)

The full turn is executed only on the forward break. It starts in the same way as the forward break half-turn, but the turn is continued to the right or clockwise with a spin on the ball of the right foot. When the dancer is again facing the original direction, the heel is dropped to stop the turning action, and a triple-time step is performed backward as "cha cha cha." The man initiates the full turn, and the woman turns on her alternate forward breaks in opposition to the man. The "get-out" is to replace the man's forward break full turn with a forward break of the basic step, and the lady follows suit by continuing her normal backward break of the basic step and omitting the full turn from her forward break. (Option—again the turning shoulder of the front dancer can be tapped by the rear dancer just before the turn.)

Suggested Sequence: (same as mambo, except substitute cha-cha) Add:

4 half-turns (complete) or the half chase

4 basic steps (complete)

4 full turns (complete) or the full chase

Suggested Musical Selections:

"Viva Tirado," El Chicano, MCA Records, MCA-60023.

"Tea for Two Cha-Cha," Tommy Dorsey, MCA Records, MCA-60015.

"Never on Sunday," Hoctor #686.

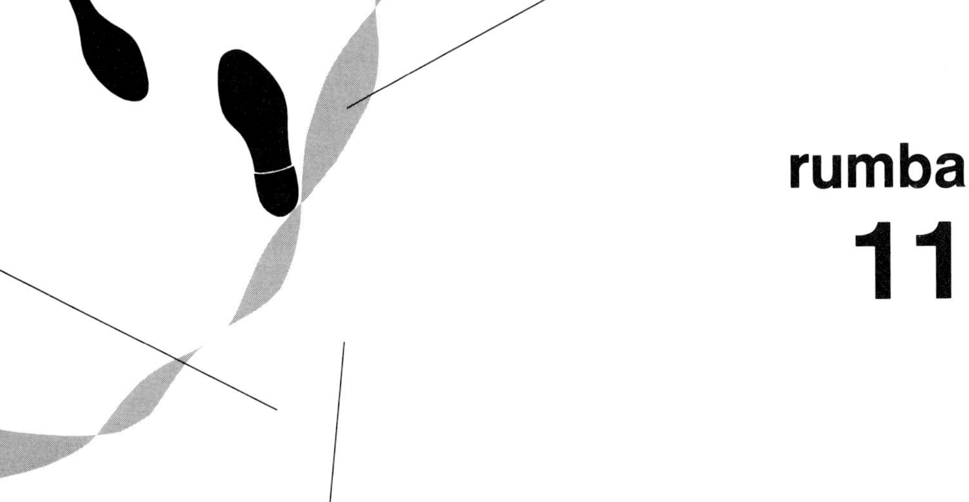

rumba
11

The rumba is the queen of the Latin rhythm dances because it was the first dance to incorporate Cuban motion. It was originally performed as an erotic dance by imported African slaves in the Caribbean, and it was refined and developed into a slower, more sentimental coquetry when introduced in the late 1920s. It created quite a sensation in the ballrooms of Europe and America because of its daring undulating rhythm of the hips. George Raft and Carole Lombard, who were American movie stars, helped to popularize the rumba.

Timing

There are two types of rumba: the Cuban rumba, which emphasizes the offbeat, and the American (square) rumba, which stresses the traditional downbeat rhythm and, as its name implies, has been adopted by America. Most rumbas are written in $\frac{4}{4}$ time but can be played either fast or slow. Americans prefer the slow version with Latin music that has a subtle, rolling quality. It is usually very melodic with background strings.

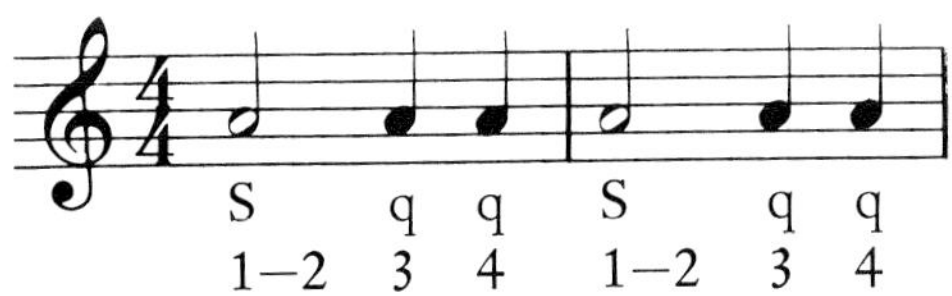

Figure 11.1. Rumba rhythmic pattern

Styling

The rumba is known for its Cuban motion styling and would be reduced to variations of a fox-trot box step without it. The student should be encouraged to practice the rolling hip motion and knee action with the footwork to perform the rumba in the correct manner. On "slow" cues, the working foot steps, unweighted, on count one, and the hip shift and weight transference occur on count two. On the "quick" cues, the same procedure occurs in one count. The cue words are "slow (shift), quick, quick" for a half box basic step.

Basic Step

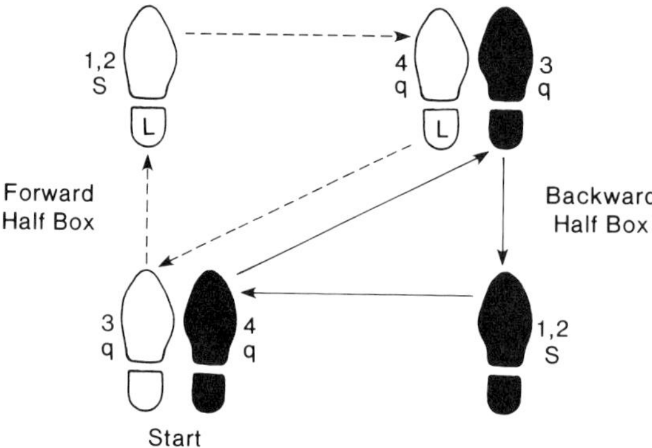

Figure 11.2. Box step, man

Step	Foot	Directional Cue	Count	Timing Cue	Comments
Forward Half Box					
1	L	Fwd	1–2	S	On ct 1, step fwd with L ft unweighted. On ct 2, shift ribcage & L hip to the L and transfer wt to L ft.
2	R	Sd	3	q	Step to R sd with R ft unweighted and immediately shift hip to R & wt to R ft.
3	L	Tog	4	q	Step to R sd with L ft unweighted and immediately shift hip to L & wt to L ft.

Step	Foot	Directional Cue	Count	Timing Cue	Comments
Backward Half Box					
1	R	Bwd	1–2	S	On ct 1, step bwd with R ft unweighted. On ct 2, shift rib-cage & R hip to the R and transfer wt to R ft.
2	L	Sd	3	q	Step to L sd with L ft unweighted and immediately shift hip to L & wt to L ft.
3	R	Tog	4	q	Step to L sd with R ft unweighted and immediately shift hip to R & wt to R ft.

Note: The man starts with the forward half box, and the woman starts with the backward half box. On count 3 of each half box, a diagonal line precedes the side step.

Variations

Progressive Step

(Man's part—similar to waltz progressive step)

Step	Foot	Directional Cue	Count	Timing Cue	Comments
Forward—2 successive Half Boxes					
1	L	Fwd	1–2	S	Cuban motion styling throughout
2	R	Sd	3	q	
3	L	Tog	4	q	
4	R	Fwd	1–2	S	
5	L	Sd	3	q	
6	R	Tog	4	q	
Backward—2 successive Half Boxes					
1	L	Bwd	1–2	S	Cuban motion styling throughout
2	R	Sd	3	q	R ft follows a diag. line to R sd.
3	L	Tog	4	q	
4	R	Bwd	1–2	S	
5	L	Sd	3	q	L ft follows a diag. line to L sd.
6	R	Tog	4	q	

Note: The Progressive Step can be performed in a series of several forward and several backward half boxes.

Step	Foot	Directional Cue	Count	Timing Cue	Comments
Woman's Part					
Forward—2 successive Half Boxes					
1	R	Bwd	1–2	S	Cuban motion styling throughout
2	L	Sd	3	q	
3	R	Tog	4	q	
4	L	Bwd	1–2	S	
5	R	Sd	3	q	
6	L	Tog	4	q	
Backward—2 successive Half Boxes					
1	R	Fwd	1–2	S	Cuban motion styling throughout
2	L	Sd	3	q	
3	R	Tog	4	q	
4	L	Fwd	1–2	S	
5	R	Sd	3	q	
6	L	Tog	4	q	

Break Variations

First Position Breaks

(Similar to the waltz balance step)

Step	Foot	Directional Cue	Count	Timing Cue	Comments
Forward					
1	L	Fwd	1–2	S	Cuban motion styling throughout (also called "hip-rises" in first pos.)
2	R	Fwd	3	q	R ft beside L ft in first pos., wt chg.
3	L	IP	4	q	Wt chg
Backward					
1	R	Bwd	1–2	S	Cuban motion styling throughout
2	L	Bwd	3	q	L ft beside R ft in first pos., wt chg.
3	R	IP	4	q	Wt chg

Note: The man starts with the forward first position break, and the woman starts with the backward first position break. They can also be performed to both sides and should be added to the forward and backward sequence.

Second Position Breaks (Man's Part)

Step	Foot	Directional Cue	Count	Timing Cue	Comments
1	L	Fwd	1–2	S	Cuban motion styling throughout
2	R	Sd	3	q	R ft follows a diag. line to R sd
3	L	IP	4	q	Second position, R ft remains to R sd
4	R	Tog	1–2	S	R ft moves beside L
5	L	Sd	3	q	L ft moves to L sd
6	R	IP	4	q	Second position, wt on R ft
Woman's Part					
1	R	Bwd	1–2	S	Cuban motion styling throughout
2	L	Sd	3	q	L ft follows a diag. line to L sd
3	R	IP	4	q	Second pos., L ft remains to L sd
4	L	Tog	1–2	S	L ft moves bsd R ft
5	R	Sd	3	q	R ft moves to R sd
6	L	IP	4	q	Second pos., wt on L ft

Fifth Position Breaks

(Similar to those in mambo)

Step	Foot	Directional Cue	Count	Timing Cue	Comments
Right Fifth Position Break					
1	L	Sd	1–2	S	Cuban motion styling throughout. Start in closed couple dance pos.
2	R	Bwd	3	q	L ft stays in place, facing fwd, while R moves bwd so that toes tch heel of L ft in 5th pos. Remaining in closed pos., turn to reverse pos. lead—L hand.
3	L	IP	4	q	
Left Fifth Position Break					
1	R	Sd	1–2	S	Cuban motion styling throughout
2	L	Bwd	3	q	R ft stays in place, facing fwd, while L moves bwd so that toes tch heel of R ft in 5th pos. Release woman's R hand from man's L to One-hand Open Pos.
3	R	IP	4	q	Lead—L hand.

Note: The man starts with the right fifth position break, and the lady starts with the left fifth position break, or, if preferred, a half basic step can precede the fifth position breaks, and the parts are reversed.

Turns

Left Box Turn

(Similar to that in fox-trot and waltz)

Step	Foot	Directional Cue	Count	Timing Cue	Comments
Forward Box Turn (¼)					
1	L	Fwd	1–2	S	Cuban motion styling throughout; arc-shaped 4th pos. fwd step with toe leading ¼ CCW turn.
2	R	Sd	3	q	R ft follows a diag. one to R sd
3	L	Tog	4	q	
Backward Box Turn (¼)					
1	R	Bwd	1–2	S	Cuban motion styling throughout; turn R ft ¼ CCW first, then body follows.
2	L	Sd	3	q	L ft follows a diag. line to L sd
3	R	Tog	4	q	

Note: Complete the full left box turn by repeating one forward and one backward box turn. The man starts with the forward box turn, and the woman starts with the backward box turn.

Underarm Turn

The man's part for the underarm turn requires the rumba box-step footwork. His lead involves the arch position with his left arm and slightly pushing the woman with his right hand to direct her under the arch. As he performs the forward half box, she walks under the arch in a small CW circle (S,q,q) and returns to face him directly to complete the box step with a forward half box.

Variation: A walk-around can be added after the woman performs an underarm turn to a full open position. The man then starts walking backward with his right foot, and the woman walks forward on her left foot in a large clockwise circle. They move simultaneously in rumba timing. To "get-out," the woman faces the man to step forward on her left, returning to the box step.

Side Pass—(Man's Part)

Step	Foot	Directional Cue	Count	Timing Cue	Comments
Forward Half Box					
1	L	Fwd	1–2	S	Cuban motion styling throughout
2	R	Sd	3	q	
3	L	Tog	4	q	

Step	Foot	Directional Cue	Count	Timing Cue	Comments
Backward Half Box (modified Left Box Turn)					
4	R	Bwd	1–2	S	Cuban motion styling throughout
5	L	Sd¼	3	q	¼ left turn on sd step and heel of R hand leads woman across in frt of him (semiopen pos.)
6	R	Tog	4	q	

Note: The woman's part is in natural opposition to the man's part except on steps 5 and 6. Step 5 involves the woman's R ft stepping straight forward to the left (across in front of the man). Step 6 consists of her L ft pivoting CCW to face directly toward the man. The sequence is then completed with the man leading a forward left box turn so that the couple is facing reverse direction of dance to continue other variations. This is a beautiful step pattern.

Suggested Sequence:

2 basic box steps (complete)

1 left box turn (complete)

4 forward progressive steps

4 backward progressive steps

4 second-position breaks (complete)

4 fifth-position breaks (complete)

4 basic box steps (complete)

1 underarm turn with walk-around variation

2 side pass variations

Suggested Musical Selections:

"Spanish Eyes," Al Martino, Starline—a subsidiary of Capitol Records, #6108.

"It's Now or Never," vocalist—Elvis Presley.

"Arrivederche Roma," Hoctor, #650.

"Adios," Hoctor, #638.

"Besame Mucho," Roper-Records, #216-A.

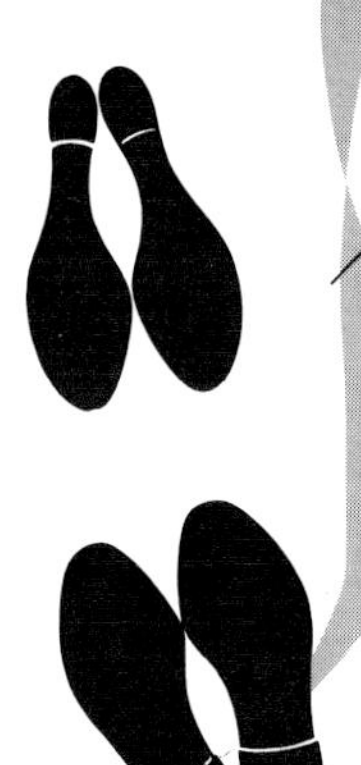

appendixes

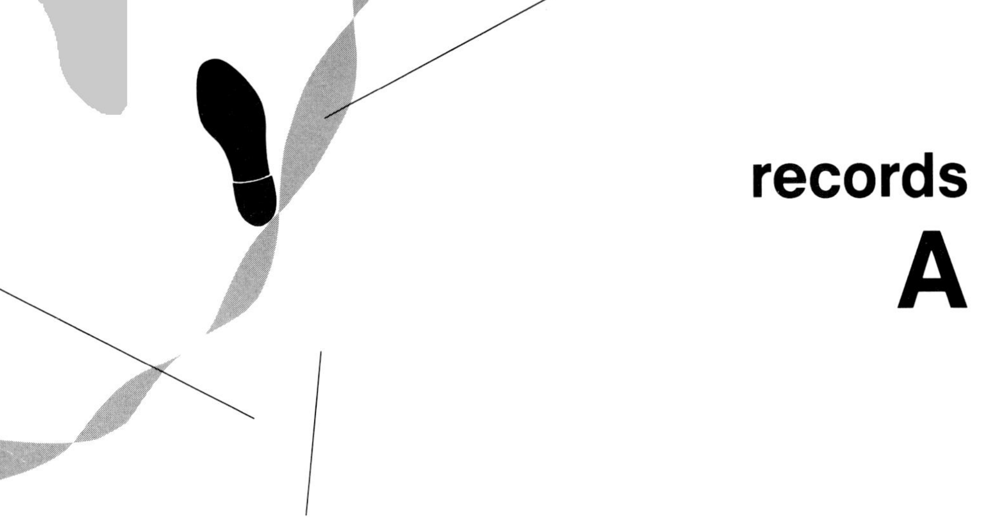

records
A

RECORD SOURCES

Most record companies will only sell directly to local dealers, who should be contacted by the social dance enthusiast for both old and new musical selections. The following companies specialize as sources of music for physical education dance classes:

Educational Activities, Inc. P.O. Box 392, Freeport, New York 11520

Educational Dance Recordings, Inc. P.O. Box 6062, Bridgeport, CT

Hoctor Educational Records, Inc., P.O. Box 38, Waldwick, New Jersey 07463
Request their 48-page brochure entitled "Ballroom Records." It includes a large selection of albums and 45-RPM records, which are each identified with a specific ballroom dance. Also request a current price list.

Kimbo Educational Records, P.O. Box 55, Deal, New Jersey 07723

Taffy's Catalog of Records and Books, 701 Beta Drive, Cleveland, OH 44143.
Request their 128-page booklet which includes a list of 45 RPM singles by title and dance identity, LP albums for ballroom dancing, etc.

Telemark Dance Records, Box 55, McLean, VA 22101
Request their ballroom dance catalogue, which includes their top 25 selling records for ballroom dancing and a variety of other types of ballroom dance albums. 45-RPM records, *Dance Week* magazine (request a free copy), and books on ballroom dancing (including formation dancing).

RECORD ALBUMS

Basic Dance Tempos. Eighteen musical selections and six dance rhythms for teaching waltz, schottische, polka, two-step, cha-cha and tango. Music is varied in tempo, and record bands are easily identifiable for teacher use.

Dance Along With Mitch. Hoctor LP 3083. Cha-cha, merengue, tango, rumba, mambo, samba are featured.

Dance Party Mixer. Music for cha-cha, polka, jitterbug and novelty dances.

Let's Dance. Hoctor LP 3067. Music for fox-trot, waltz, lindy, rumba, tango, cha-cha.

How To Dance. Prepared by Betty White, professional dance instructor and author of *Dancing Made Easy*. The emphasis is on rapid learning through enthusiastic participation. Illustrated instruction manual included. D-101 fox-trot, D-102 waltz, D-103 cha-cha, D-104 rumba, D-105 samba, D-106 tango, D-107 Charleston, D-108 polka, D-109 lindy, D-110 merengue/samba.

Arthur Murray's Music for Dancing. RCA-Victor LPM 1909. (Located in Camden, NJ) Selected music for the fox-trot, waltz, tango, swing, samba, merengue, mambo, cha-cha, rumba.

Social Dancing Made Easy. A series of records prepared by Ted Nicholas, Director of Physical Education at High Plain School, Orange, CN. Each record contains five or more lessons with verbal instructions. Provision is also made for continuous dancing. Series of ten records: fox-trot, waltz, Argentine tango, jitterbug, polka, samba, merengue, mambo, cha-cha, rumba.

The Standard Thirteen for Dancing. Roper RLP 1007A. (43–48 48th St., Long Island City, NY) Fox-trot, waltz, swing, polka music.

VIDEO CASSETTE TAPE

Social Dance. Specifically produced to accompany this text. See Preface.

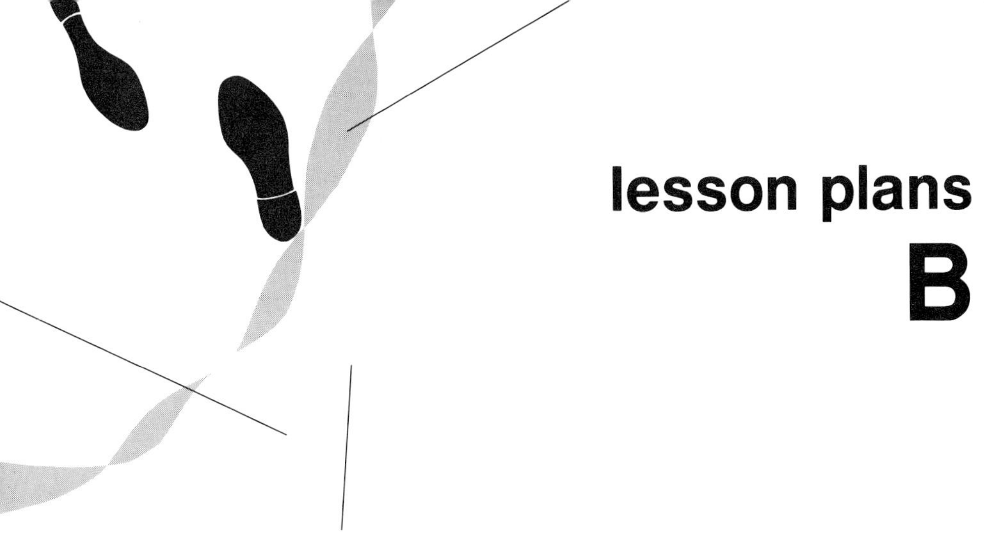

lesson plans B

Minimum
Contact Hrs.

1	Review pertinent information in chapter 1 and assign readings.
1	Introduce smooth dances. Cover brief history of fox-trot. Inform students of fox-trot timing and styling. Demonstrate, explain and render individual assistance on the man's and woman's parts of the box step, magic step (forward and backward). Switch partners.
1	Swing step, dip, conversation step.
1	Magic left turn with variations, left box turn.
1	Pivot turns and add suggested sequence.
1	Practice sequence.
1	Cover brief history of waltz. Inform students of waltz timing and styling. Demonstrate, explain and render individual assistance on the man's and woman's parts of the box step, hesitation and balance, progressive step (forward and backward), left box turn, hesitation and left box turn with cross variation, underarm turn. Add suggested sequence.
1	Review fox-trot and waltz. Cover brief history of tango. Inform students of tango timing and styling. Demonstrate, explain and render individual assistance on the man's and woman's parts of the basic step (forward and backward), quarter turn and cross variation, conversation step, medio corté, la puerta. If time and skill level permit, add butterfly fan step. Add sequence.

1   Review smooth dances and skill test on one or more of them. (Classroom space can be divided so that skill test participants and other class members who wish to practice are separated. Test can be administered before or after instructional phases.)

1   Introduce rhythm dances. Cover brief history of swing. Inform students of swing timing and styling. Demonstrate, explain and render individual assistance on the man's and woman's parts of single-time, double-time, triple-time, turning basic

1   throw-out, underarm turn and exchange, tuck underarm turn, hand-push tuck turn.

1   Equivalents, West Coast swing basic, lindy basic, shag basic. Add suggested sequence.

1   Cover polka background, timing and styling. Teach basic step, turning basic, forward basic, heel-and-toe polka. Add sequence.

1   Add similar regional dances (schottische, two-step, cotton-eyed Joe).

1   Introduce Latin rhythm dances. Discuss samba background, timing and styling. Teach basic step (attempting rise and fall), left box turn, chassé, copacabana. Add suggested sequence.

1   Discuss merengue background, timing and styling. Teach basic step (forward and backward), box step and combinations, left box turn, underarm turn, circle turn. Add suggested sequence.

1   Introduce the Cuban dances and attempt Cuban motion. Cover mambo background, timing and styling. Teach basic step, open break, crossover breaks, fifth-position breaks, parallel breaks. Add suggested sequence.

1   Review cha-cha background, timing and styling. Teach basic step and other breaks (interrelate with mambo), half turn (half chase) and full turn (full chase). Add suggested sequence.

1   Rumba background, timing and styling are compared to other Cuban dances. Teach basic box step, progressive step, second- and fifth-position breaks, left box turn, underarm turns, side pass. Add sequence. (Review rhythm dances and skill test.)

1   Written test for course. (Suggestion: include a few questions in which musical recordings are played and matched to specific dances.) Social dance teachers can contact author for example of written exam. Fee for service, postage and handling is $5. Zip code is 62026.

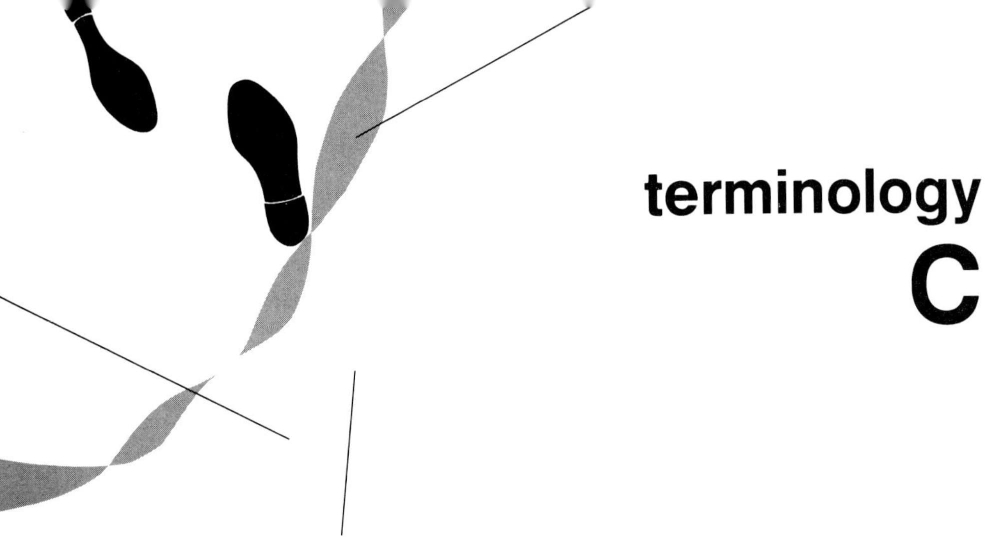

terminology
C

Brush—The ball of the foot lightly touches the floor as it passes the weighted foot.

Chassé—A sideward pattern of steps in which the free foot does not pass the weighted foot.

Close—A transfer of weight as the feet are brought together, side-by-side.

Contrabody movement—An advanced styling technique, especially on turns, in which opposition in movement of the dancer's body parts is stressed.

Cross—The free foot is moved sideward to pass in front of or behind the weighted foot.

Direction of dance—The movement of dancers in a counter-clockwise direction around the dance floor.

Draw—A slow, gradual sideward step in which there is no weight change.

Follow-through   Continuous movement in the same direction.

"Get-out"—Completing the variation to return to the original position.

Hop—Projecting the body upward so that the take-off foot and the landing foot are the same.

In place—A weight change involving no directional motion.

Kick—A directional lift of the free foot with no weight change. The toes are usually pointed.

Lead—A man's method of indicating the next step to his partner.

Pivot—A turn on the ball of the foot.

Point—The toes and ankle form a straight line with the leg.

Quick—Short steps that require one count.

Reverse direction of dance—The movement of dancers in a clockwise direction around the dance floor.

Rise and fall—An "up-and-down" style of movement in specific dances.

109

Rock—A transference of weight from one foot to the other without altering the foot position.

Slow—Long steps that require two counts.

Supporting leg—The leg carrying the body weight.

"Sweeping turn"—The left foot describes an arc-shaped ¼ turn, forward in 4th position.

"T-turn"—The right foot turns ¼ backward (CCW) so that the toes point toward the heel of the left foot which (momentarily) points straight ahead. It could be called "inverted fifth position," but a wider stance is encouraged.

Touch—The free foot makes contact with the floor without changing weight.

Working leg—The moving leg.

"W" position—The arms are held sideward, forming a "W," to assimilate the basic closed dance position.

Weight change—Transferring body weight from one foot to the other foot.

bibliography

Astaire, Fred, and Engle, Lyle K. *The Fred Astaire Dance Book.* MO: Cornerstone Press, 1962.

Barrows, Frank. *Latin American Dancing.* London: Frederick Muller Ltd., 1964.

Buckman, Peter. *Let's Dance.* New York, London: Paddington Press Ltd., 1978.

Dow, Allen. *The Official Guide to Ballroom Dancing.* Northbrook, IL: Domus Books, 1980.

Ellfeldt, Lois, and Morton, Virgil L. *This is Ballroom Dance.* Palo Alto, CA: National Press Books, 1974.

Fallon, Dennis, J., and Kuchenmeister, Sue Ann. *The Art of Ballroom Dance.* Minneapolis, MN: Burgess Publishing Co., 1977.

Ford, Henry and Mrs. *Good Morning.* Dearborn, MI: The Dearborn Publishing Co., 1926.

Heaton, Alma. *Social Dance Rhythms.* Provo, Utah: Brigham University Press, 1978.

Harris, Jane A., Pittman and Waller. *Dance Awhile.* Minneapolis, MN: Burgess Publishing Co., 5th ed., 1978.

Kraus, Richard. *History of the Dance in Art and Education.* Englewood Cliffs, NJ: Prentice Hall, Inc., 1950.

Kraus, Richard, and Sadlo, Lola. *Beginning Social Dance.* Belmont, CA: Wadsworth Publishing Co, Inc., 1964.

Livingston, Peter. *Country Swing and Western Dance.* Garden City, NY: Doubleday and Co., Inc., 1981.

Murray, Arthur. *How To Become a Good Dancer.* NY: Pocket Books, 1976.

Pillach, William F. *Social Dance.* (Physical Education Activities Series). Dubuque, IA: Wm. C. Brown Publishers, 1967.

Silvester, Victor. *Modern Ballroom Dancing.* London: Barrie & Jenkins, Ltd. 1977.

Villacorta, Aurora. *Step by Step to Ballroom Dancing.* Danville, IL: The Interstate Printers & Publishers, Inc., 1974.

Youmans, J. *Social Dance.* Pacific Palisades, CA: Goodyear Publishing Co., Inc., 1969.

index

References to illustrations are printed in boldface.